Color Atlas of Dermatology

Frieboes/Schönfeld

Color Atlas of Dermatology

by

Joseph Kimmig, M.D.

Professor of Dermatology, Chief of the Department of Dermatology and the
Dispensary, University Hospital, Hamburg

and

Michael Jänner, M.D.

Research Assistant, Department of Dermatology and Dispensary, University
Hospital, Hamburg

with 927 Figures, Mostly in Color

American Edition Translated and Revised by

Herbert Goldschmidt, M.D.

Assistant Professor of Clinical Dermatology,
University of Pennsylvania School of Medicine

With a Foreword to the American Edition by

Donald M. Pillsbury, M.D.

Professor and Former Chairman of the Department of Dermatology,
University of Pennsylvania School of Medicine

W. B. Saunders Company · Philadelphia & London

Printed in Germany

Title of the original German Edition: FRIEBOES/SCHOENFELD, Atlas der Haut- und Geschlechtskrank-
heiten, 3. neubearbeitete Auflage, fortgeführt von J. KIMMIG und M. JÄNNER, Georg Thieme Verlag,
Stuttgart

English translation published by W. B. Saunders Company, Philadelphia and London, 1966
Library of Congress catalog card number 66 - 16 253
Reprinted May, 1967

FOREWORD

Of all the organ systems of the human body, the skin obviously is the one most suited to photographic or other illustrative methods of demonstrating the disease states to which it is susceptible.

With the marked increase in recent years in knowledge of the precise cutaneous and systemic backgrounds of many diseases affecting the skin, and significant advances in the technology of color photography, illustration of dermatologic diseases has increased in fidelity and impact. Such records of disease have become extraordinarily faithful to the living state, and occupy an essential place in teaching and clinical research. It is believed that even the most cursory examination of the FRIEBOES-SCHÖNFELD Atlas will impress the viewer with this fact. Pictures of the common diseases of the skin are recognizable in a flash, and those of less common ones provide all the necessary visible clues. The explanatory text has been amended and expanded in the translation by Dr. GOLDSCHMIDT.

The history of this Atlas is of interest because it is a record of a proud influential school of dermatology which largely disintegrated during World War II, but then rose from the ashes to its previous place of eminence in world dermatology and medicine. Frieboes was the original collector of the photographs, beginning in 1941. He assembled some three-quarters of the illustrations in the first edition by 1949, a remarkable achievement, but died before writing the text. SCHÖNFELD completed the task of publication. The present edition by KIMMIG and JÄNNER is a completely new book; with but a few exceptions all of the illustrations of the first and second editions have been replaced, and their number more than doubled. None of the previous text has been used. But true to German standards of personal and academic loyalty, the names of the original authors have been deservedly perpetuated and honored.

Preparation and publication of an atlas of this size entirely in the U.S.A. could result only in financial disaster to the publisher. The American publishers have performed a distinct service in making it available in English. The translator, indeed more properly the American co-author, has brought an extensive background of training and accomplishment in both Germany and the U.S.A. to his task, and will be justly rewarded by the thanks of all students and physicians who benefit from this impressive volume.

DONALD M. PILLSBURY, M. D.

PREFACE TO THE THIRD EDITION

The third edition of the Color Atlas of Dermatology is based on clinical records of the Department of Dermatology, University of Hamburg. Technical advances in the field of color reproduction have enabled us to give the Atlas a completely new face. Some material from the second edition has been included, e.g., illustrations of venereal diseases and of some rare dermatologic disorders. We are also indebted to Dr. K. F. Schaller and Dr. W. Müller of Hamburg, and to Prof. G. Bopp of Porto Alegre, who contributed valuable material on leprosy, yaws, leishmaniasis, and tropical skin diseases.

Work on this Atlas was greatly aided by the excellent cooperation and vast experience of the Georg Thieme Verlag under the direction of Mr. Günther Hauff. Our thanks are due also to the engraving house of Brend'Amour, Simhart & Co., Munich, for careful and accurate reproduction of the photographs.

The Atlas of Dermatology, inaugurated by E. Frieboes and W. Schönfeld, is intended to be used in conjunction with one of the current textbooks of dermatology; we hope that it will aid medical students, general practitioners, internists, and dermatologists in the recognition of dermatologic disorders.

Joseph Kimmig, M. D.

Michael Jänner, M. D.

CONTENTS

Macular Eruptions

Erythemas

Erythema, the most common reaction of the skin, is due to dilatation of the capillaries (hyperemia). The affected skin blanches momentarily on diascopic examination with a glass slide, but the redness reappears as soon as the pressure is relieved. A variety of causes may be responsible for active (inflammatory) or passive (stasis) hyperemia.

Erythema may be localized or widespread, ranging from minute macules to involvement of the entire body surface, as in erythrodermas. According to their configuration, the patches are classified as annular, gyrate, circinate, or serpiginous erythemas. Macules covering the entire integument in regular distribution are often called exanthemata. The following disorders are associated with a classic monomorphous erythematous or exanthematous eruption: scarlet fever, measles, German measles, certain types of dermatitis, erythema infectiosum, erythema chronicum migrans, and scarlatiniform and morbilliform drug eruptions. Some of these disorders will be discussed elsewhere.

When active hyperemia is followed by edema, extravasation, and infiltration, the erythema may assume a polymorphous appearance of urticarial, vesicular, hemorrhagic, or papular character. A good example is erythema infectiosum variabile, a relatively new entity.

Erythema infectiosum variabile
(Margarine disease)

An epidemic erythematous eruption involving thousands of patients was observed in Germany and Holland in 1958 and 1959. The exanthema appeared on the proximal parts of the extremities and sometimes on the face, usually without prodromal manifestations, and spread rapidly over the entire integument. It was accompanied by severe itching and, in rare cases, by elevated temperatures. A wide variety of eruptions was seen, particularly erythema multiforme-like lesions, and mor-

billiform and papular eruptions. Vesicular and hemorrhagic changes were observed less frequently. On the fourth or fifth day after its onset, the exanthema began to regress and the itching subsided.

Although a viral etiology could not be ruled out, many authors believe that this protean eruption was caused by a new emulsifier used in the production of margarine in those countries. Peculiarly, the highest incidence of the disease was seen in young female adults; children under 10 years were practically never affected.

Erythema chronicum migrans
(Lipschütz and Afzelius)

This disease usually starts with red macules, which develop into ringed erythematous lesions with light red, only slightly raised migrating margins and pale or livid centers. In some cases the eruption seems to follow insect bites, especially tick bites. Viruses or toxins contained in tick saliva have been discussed as etiologic agents. This disorder is extremely rare on the American continent.

Ulerythema ophryogenes (Unna and Taenzer)

A variant of keratosis pilaris, this disorder affects the eyebrows from where it may spread to the forehead and cheeks. The skin shows a persistent reticulated erythema with small follicular horny papules and, in some instances, fine scaling. This rare condition culminates in atrophy and loss of hair in the affected areas.

Erythema multiforme (von Hebra)
(Erythema exudativum multiforme)

The classic, idiopathic erythema multiforme is characterized by symmetrical, bright bluish red to dark purple, slightly infiltrated, round macules with a tendency to spread peripherally. These lesions are found on the dorsal aspects of hands, fingers, feet, and toes, and on the adjacent areas of the extremities. They may or may not be accompanied by systemic symptoms. In the initial stage, the central portion of the lesions usually shows a bluish-gray discoloration, which is intensified during the next few days; simultaneously, a central depression develops. As a rule, the polymorphous lesions subside completely after a few more days.

In other cases, the disorder may manifest itself in concentric rings (target or iris lesions), or in peculiar circinate lesions with peripheral rings and central disks showing a lighter color than the midzone. Other variants are characterized by large blisters (bullous erythema multiforme), which may contain a hemorrhagic exudate.

A variant affecting predominantly the palms and soles is referred to as the "inverse type." Confluent lesions, especially on the palms, result in edematous, livid, pernio-like skin changes. In the form of large blisters, the disease may also affect the buccal mucosa, sometimes in combination with the cutaneous changes described above. In some cases, especially in male patients, the genitals may become involved. In its severe, sometimes fatal generalized form, the disease is often classified as STEVENS-JOHNSON syndrome. It affects mostly children and young adults and starts with high fever, malaise and severe stomatitis, conjunctivitis, urethritis, and balanitis, followed later by the typical skin lesions of erythema multiforme.

Despite its characteristic morphology, erythema multiforme is not an etiologic entity but a reaction pattern.

The *idiopathic form* of the disease is probably of viral etiology. Herpes simplex labialis frequently precedes the onset of this type, which often has a seasonal incidence (spring or fall).

Symptomatic forms, closely resembling the idiopathic type in their morphology, may be due to internal medication (salicylates, sulfonamides, hydantoin derivatives, phenacetin, barbiturates, iodides, bromides) or may follow systemic diseases (bacterial or viral infections, allergic disorders, malignancies). The symptomatic form of erythema multiforme seldom involves the buccal mucosa; typical iris lesions are rare. Diagnosis is based on history and clinical course of the disease. Differentiation between gyrate forms of erythema multiforme and urticaria is particularly difficult. (Urticaria is characterized by pruritus and evanes-

cence of the eruption.) When the oral mucosa is involved, differential diagnosis includes bullous drug eruptions, pemphigus, and dermatitis herpetiformis. Syphilis must be ruled out when the lesions are confined to the genitals.

Erythema nodosum (VON HEBRA)

This syndrome is characterized by successive crops of symmetrical, bright red, tender nodules with smooth surface, varying in size from 1 to 5 cm., and occasionally coalescing to form large indurations on the lower extremities. Vascular damage may lead to extravasation of blood and, due to degradation of hemoglobin, to greenish or bluish-yellow purpuric discolorations (contusiform type of erythema nodosum). Ulceration is extremely rare. Predilection sites are the anterior surfaces of the lower legs, less often those of the thighs. At times, the extensor surfaces of the arms may be affected. The disease is self-limited and occurs chiefly in young adults. Recurrent and seasonal forms are not rare. The attacks are often associated with mild constitutional symptoms such as malaise, fever, and pains in muscles and joints.

Differential diagnosis includes erythema induratum (BAZIN), insect bites, drug eruptions, and periarteritis nodosa. Symptomatic forms include nodular cutaneous reactions associated with infectious diseases, particularly streptococcal infections (scarlet fever, rheumatic fever), fungal infections (coccidioidomycosis), tuberculosis (in children), leprosy, chicken pox, lymphogranuloma venereum, and syphilis. The erythema nodosum reaction pattern can also be elicited by drugs (iodides, bromides, sulfonamides, penicillin). It also can be seen in sarcoidosis.

Erythema elevatum diutinum
(CROCKER and WILLIAMS)

The pathogenesis and etiology of this rare disorder are uncertain. Erythema elevatum diutinum is slightly painful and shows a preference for the hands and the extensor surfaces of the extremities, especially about the joints of the fingers, wrists, elbows and knees. The characteristic lesions are elevated round, oval or polygonal nodules, 0.5 to 2 cm. in diameter, often in annular arrangement; their color varies from red to purple. Their surface is smooth, sometimes showing central depression. The oral mucosa is not involved; general health is not impaired. The lesions may persist for many months. Differential diagnosis includes granuloma annulare (which it resembles closely clinically) and erythema multiforme. Some authors consider erythema elevatum diutinum a variant of the latter disorder.

Toxic epidermal necrolysis (LYELL)

This grave, often fatal syndrome has an acute onset with localized or disseminated erythematous lesions. Advanced stages are characterized by large flaccid blisters. The epidermis sloughs off in large sheets as in a widespread scalding burn, leaving a moist, dark red, raw dermal surface. The disease is associated with fever and severe systemic manifestations; the mucous membranes are often involved. In many cases the disorder is caused by allergic or toxic drug reactions (e.g., to sulfonamides, hydantoin, antipyrine). Severe erythema multiforme (STEVENS-JOHNSON syndrome) and epidermolysis bullosa may present similar cutaneous lesions.

Erythema annulare rheumaticum
(LEHNDORF and LEINER)

Pale red to livid rings, 2 to 4 mm. in diameter appear, and either break up or form polycyclic configurations. This disease occurs exclusively in children with acute rheumatic fever associated with endocarditis or pericarditis. Preferred areas are the chest, abdomen, back, and thighs.

Erythema annulare centrifugum (DARIER)

This syndrome has an abrupt onset but usually runs a chronic, often recurrent course; its cause is unknown. An initial erythema develops into a large wheal, which rapidly grows eccentrically with a raised urticarial border, while the central portion returns to the level of the surrounding normal skin, leaving a yellowish or faintly pigmented, slightly scaling surface. Polycyclic and gyrate configurations are frequently seen. In the course of several weeks, new lesions replace the old ones. The disease predominantly affects adults, involving primarily the trunk and the proximal portions of the extremities. Similar eruptions have been described as autoimmune reactions, dermatophytids (trichophytin test),

and in association with rheumatoid arthritis and internal malignant tumors.

Purpura

Morphologically, three main varieties of purpura are described. Petechiae are superficial hemorrhagic macules that are round, 1 to 5 mm. in diameter, and sharply outlined. Ecchymoses are slightly deeper and more extensive round or irregular extravasations. Hematomas are large, deep bluish, rounded, poorly outlined fluctuant collections of extravasated blood.

Cutaneous hemorrhages are not a disease entity. Unlike erythematous eruptions, extravasations of blood (hemosiderin) into the skin cannot be blanched by diascopy (firm pressure with a glass slide). Exanthematous patterns of blood extravasations into the skin are described clinically as *purpura*, a term indicating neither cause nor adequate treatment of this hemorrhagic disorder. Some forms of purpura are entirely benign, whereas others may signify extremely serious diseases. Clinical and laboratory tests permit differentiation of: (1) purpura with coagulation defects; (2) purpura with thrombocytic defects (thrombocytopenia, thrombasthenia); and (3) purpura with vascular damage (damage to the capillary endothelium due to hypoxemia, allergic reactions, or vitamin deficiency).

Purpura with coagulation defects is often induced by trauma (e.g., hemophilia), while in the case of thrombopenic and vascular purpura, petechiae appear spontaneously or without visible traumatization.

Purpura with coagulation defects

Hyperglobulinemic purpura (WALDENSTRØM)

Hypergammaglobulinemia, resulting in a shift in the ratio of normal plasma protein fractions (dysproteinemia), and vascular changes lead to hemorrhages into skin and mucous membranes. The disease takes a recurrent course and has a favorable prognosis.

Other common causes of purpura due to coagulation defects are *prothrombin deficiency* (congenital, vitamin K deficiency, hepatic disorders), *fibrinogen deficiency, hemophilia,* and *anticoagulant drugs.*

Purpura with thrombocytic defects

Idiopathic thrombocytopenic purpura
(WERLHOF)

Petechiae or ecchymoses, usually of a pronounced purple or bluish color, are characteristic of this disorder. Diagnosis is based on blood tests, an episodic course, hemorrhages into the mucous membranes, internal hemorrhages, higher incidence in young females than in males, splenomegaly, and positive RUMPEL-LEEDE sign. The acute allergic form often follows infections, shows massive purpuric lesions, and is usually self-limited. The chronic form has a gradual onset and a long history of easy bruising and bleeding of mucous membranes, frequently with gastrointestinal hemorrhages; typical cutaneous purpura is less common.

Purpuric eruptions are also seen in *hereditary hemorrhagic thrombasthenia* (GLANZMANN), in *constitutional thrombopathy* (VON WILLEBRAND-JÜRGENS) and in *thrombotic thrombocytopenic purpura*.

Symptomatic thrombocytopenia

The symptomatic thrombocytopenias are of great clinical importance. Severe toxic infections (septicemia, scarlet fever, virus infections, tuberculosis), tumors with bone marrow metastases, leukemia, hypersplenism, pancytopenia, radiation damage, and drug reactions (quinine, diphenylhydantoin, sulfonamides, salicylates) are frequently associated with marked thrombocytopenia leading to cutaneous and mucosal hemorrhages.

Purpura with vascular damage

The common criterion of this rather heterogeneous group is vascular damage; defects in coagulation factors and platelets are less important. The principal pathogenetic factors are vitamin C deficiency and disturbance of vitamin C utilization in the case of *scurvy*; degenerative changes of the vascular walls and surrounding connective tissue in the case of *senile purpura*; and increased hydrostatic pressure resulting in breakage of capillary walls in the case of *stasis purpura* and the pigmented purpuric eruptions of MAJOCCHI's, SCHAMBERG's, and

GOUGEROT-BLUM's diseases. These latter entities are probably the same disease with slightly different morphology.

Purpura annularis telangiectodes (MAJOCCHI)

In this disease symmetrically arranged, pink telangiectatic punctae develop into small macular hemorrhages of reddish-brown coloration, usually on the lower legs. Ring-like configurations may occur, and central atrophy may develop in extensive lesions. The disease causes no appreciable discomfort. In patients with high blood pressure, the purpuric changes are due to functional peripheral vasoconstriction and vascular damage. The incidence of the disease is highest in middle-aged males.

Progressive pigmentary dermatosis
(SCHAMBERG)

This syndrome, which also is more common in middle-aged men, probably represents a variant of the purpura described above. Ring formations are absent. Predominant features are poorly outlined brownish-yellow or reddish patches of varying size, with peripheral punctate petechiae; the color is described as resembling cayenne pepper. Differential diagnosis includes drug eruptions.

Pigmented purpuric lichenoid dermatitis
(GOUGEROT-BLUM)

The eruption usually involves the lower extremities (rarely the trunk), is often pruritic, and resembles SCHAMBERG's disease. It is characterized by lichenoid, polygonal, flat-topped, slightly elevated purpuric papules densely grouped within brownish plaques. The papules later assume a bluish to brownish-red tinge — "embedded grains of paprika."

Schönlein's purpura

This hemorrhagic syndrome is also known as allergic, anaphylactoid, or rheumatic purpura, or as a form of allergic vasculitis. Joint involvement is part of its symptomatology, yet its pathogenesis and pathologic anatomy are quite distinct from those of rheumatic fever. The eruption is often preceded by an infectious disease. Food and drug allergies must be ruled out.

The symmetrically arranged exanthema occurs mostly in children, showing a preference for the extensor surfaces of the legs. In severe cases, it may involve the entire integument, with the exception of popliteal and antecubital areas, palms, soles and face. The lesions may range from discrete, pinhead to dime sized, pale red spots to dark red wheals or hemorrhagic vesicles. Synovitis and gastrointestinal symptoms (vomiting, colicky pains, intestinal hemorrhages) may aggravate the condition. This abdominal form is also called Schönlein-Henoch *purpura* or *purpura abdominalis* Henoch.

Purpura fulminans

This very severe, usually fatal type of purpura occurs mostly in children. The disease follows an infection and takes a rapidly progressive course resembling a Sanarelli-Shwartzman phenomenon. The preceding fulminating septicemia is often caused by Neisseria meningitidis, Streptococcus hemolyticus or Pseudomonas aeruginosa. Hemorrhages also occur in internal organs, particularly in the adrenal glands (Waterhouse-Friderichsen syndrome).

Triple syndrome of Gougerot

The three characteristic features of this febrile dermatosis are annular erythematous or papular skin lesions, ranging in size from 0.2 to 2.0 cm.; small macular, disseminated purpura; and minute to lentil-sized, tender subcutaneous nodules. The disorder is considered an allergic reaction induced by an infectious disease.

Disturbances of Pigmentation

In addition to erythematous eruptions (due to dilated vessels) and purpuric lesions due to extravasation of blood cells, macular skin changes can also be caused by endogenous or exogenous pigments. The most important pigments causing such changes are melanin, lipofuscin, and hemosiderin.

Common variants of pigmentation due to melanin are *freckles, lentigines*, and *pigmented nevi;* they are only of cosmetic importance. Premalignant lesions are rare.

The *blue nevus* (nevus caeruleus) is characterized by the presence of melanocytes in the corium, as is the *Mongolian spot*. The blue nevus usually occurs singly, is sharply demarcated and not more than lentil-sized. Malignant degeneration (melanosarcoma) is very rare.

Pigmentation-polyposis syndrome (Peutz-Jeghers)

Discrete, dark brown to black pigmented macules of irregular configuration are located about the mouth, on the oral mucosa, around the nostrils and eyes, and on the fingers and toes. The disease usually occurs before the third decade and shows a high familial incidence. A thorough examination of the intestinal tract is indicated, since the skin lesions are often associated with polyposis, usually of the small intestine (abdominal pain and bleeding). Malignant degeneration of the polyps is very rare (in contrast to the potentially malignant familial polyposis of the large bowel).

Chloasma

Chloasma uterinum may occur during pregnancy (on the face, linea alba, areolae of nipples, genitals). *Chloasma extrauterinum* is seen in menopausal women (on the lateral aspects of neck) following therapy with female hormones, or in the presence of ovarian tumors. *Chloasma virginum* (located periorally) may affect adolescent girls and young women with dysmenorrhea. Patients with hepatic disorders occasionally show periocular hyperpigmentation.

Incontinentia pigmenti (Bloch-Sulzberger)

Irregularly shaped, linear, or gyrate pigmented lesions of brown to grayish-brown color develop in early infancy, predominantly in female patients. This type of pigmentation is probably postinflammatory; it is preceded by erythematous, urticarial or vesicular changes and may be associated with neurologic and osseous defects.

Postinflammatory pigmentation

Hyperpigmentation due to increased melanin formation is associated with a number of inflammatory dermatoses (postinflammatory pigmentation). Lichen planus, neurodermatitis, and fixed drug eruptions have a pronounced tendency to produce such changes.

Caloric stimuli may produce *melanoderma reticularis calorica* (livedo reticularis e calore). Chemical and actinic damage also may cause hyperpigmentation. The use of photosensitizers, such as eau de cologne or oil of bergamot, followed by exposure to solar radiation, may result in *berloque dermatitis*.

Riehl's melanosis and melanodermatitis toxica (HOFFMANN)

These two syndromes are probably identical. Contact with industrial lubricants, exposure to fumes of melted tar, and prolonged cosmetic use of Vaseline or other petrolatum products may produce these changes. One of the most common macular hyperpigmentations of this type is *vaselinoderma*, usually observed about the face in women.

Arsenical melanosis

Slate-colored macular melanoderma can be traced frequently to prolonged administration of arsenicals, especially in the treatment of psoriasis vulgaris (FOWLER's solution and similar preparations). The characteristic tone of the discoloration is due to true hyperpigmentation as well as to deposits of metallic arsenic in the skin. Hyperkeratoses and squamous cell epitheliomas also may result from the use of arsenicals.

Hyperpigmentation associated with vitamin deficiency, hormonal imbalance, or endogenous and exogenous pigments

Reddish-brown, sharply defined erythemas on the face, neck, and dorsa of the hands (i.e., light-exposed areas) are characteristic of *pellagra* and *pellagroids*. These disorders are due to dietary deficiency or malabsorption of nicotinic acid amide (PP-factor).

In ADDISON's *disease*, yellowish to dark brown hyperpigmentation occurs in exposed skin areas, as well as in pressure areas, scar tissue, and the buccal mucosa; in the latter location, the lesions have a bluish-gray tone. The hyperpigmentation is due to hormonal factors.

The generalized diffuse, grayish-brown, bronze-like pigmentation seen in *hemochromatosis* (bronze diabetes) is due to hemosiderin deposits and increased melanin formation.

Typical discolorations may be produced by bile pigments (*icterus*), Atabrine, carotene (*carotenosis*), silver (*argyria*), bismuth, or gold (*chrysiasis*).

Powder stains and *tattoo marks* are caused by the accidental or intentional introduction of foreign bodies (coal dust, metal particles, powder, soot, indigo, carmine, India ink, vermilion) into the skin.

Achromia

Nevus achromicus (congenital pigmentary deficiency) and *nevus anemicus* (hypoplasia or aplasia of superficial blood vessels) manifest themselves as white patches.

Vitiligo

Discrete or multiple white patches, appearing gradually or in successive spurts, produce the picture of vitiligo. This hypopigmentation may occur in any age group. Its cause is unknown; melanocytes are present. The most common areas are the anogenital region, face, hands, and neck. The hair also may become white. The borders of the surrounding normal skin sometimes show hyperpigmentation; the edges are usually convex.

Leukoderma acquisitum centrifugum (SUTTON)

Also known as *halo nevus* or *perinevoid vitiligo*, this disorder is frequently associated with vitiligo. A pigmented nevus is surrounded by a depigmented halo. In some cases, the pigmented nevus later disappears spontaneously.

Leukoderma

Acquired types of depigmentation of known etiology are often called leukodermas. The most common type is *postinflammatory leukoderma*. Patchy depigmentation due to inhibition of melanin production may occur following such inflammatory dermatoses as syphilis, leprosy, pinta, or psoriasis. *Occupational leukoderma* is often caused by rubber or other products containing hydroquinone.

Pseudoleukodermas are due to deposits on the skin surface (fungus growth, scales) that shield the affected areas from UV-radiation and thus interfere with normal pigmentation.

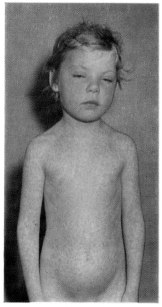

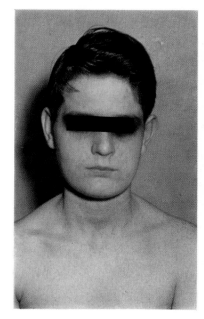

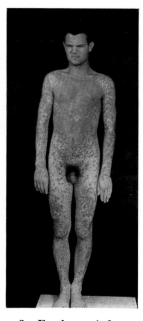

1 Measles (rubeola)

Small, round or oval, reddish-brown, partially coalescing macules disseminated over the entire body surface. Photophobia.

2 German measles (rubella)

Small, round or oval, pink, noncoalescing maculopapular lesions of varying size. Individual lesions are usually larger than in scarlet fever, and smaller than in measles. Occipital, cervical and postauricular lymphadenopathy.

3 Erythema infectiosum variabile (infectious exanthema)

Small, dusky red erythematous macules distributed over the entire integument, including scalp, palms, and soles.

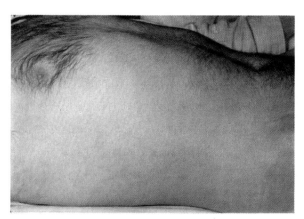

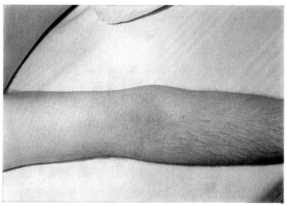

4 Scarlet fever (scarlatina)

Diffuse pink-red flush of the skin with punctate (goose-flesh) papular lesions. The rash is best seen in intertriginous areas.

5 Positive Rumpel-Leede test in scarlet fever

Petechial hemorrhages in the antecubital area following application of a tourniquet. This test is often positive in scarlet fever.

8

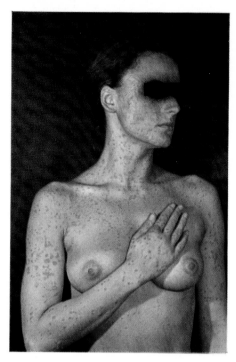

6 Erythema infectiosum variabile
Dark red macular eruption disseminated over entire body surface.

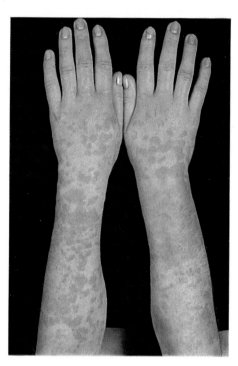

7 Erythema infectiosum variabile
Erythema multiforme-like eruption of forearms. Discrete and coalescent erythematous lesions.

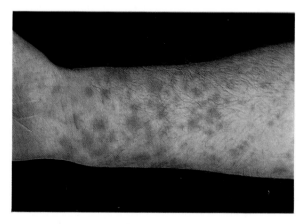

8 Erythema infectiosum variabile
Erythema multiforme-like partially hemorrhagic lesions on the flexor aspect of the forearm.

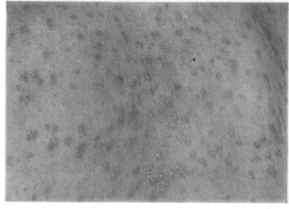

9 Erythema infectiosum variabile
Maculovesicular lesions on the back.

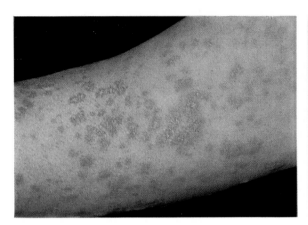

10 Erythema infectiosum variabile
Maculovesicular eruption on the thigh.

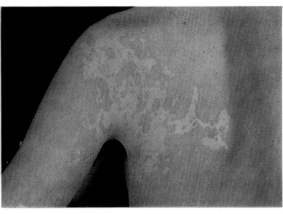

11 Erythema infectiosum variabile
Large confluent erythematous patches with islands of normal skin.

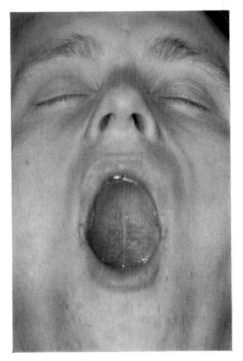

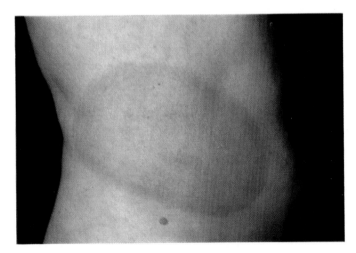

12 Erythema infectiosum variabile
Discrete and coalescent erythematous mucosal lesions (enanthema).

13 Erythema chronicum migrans (Lipschütz)
Large, oval, pale livid plaque with band-like pink raised migrating border, probably originating from a tick bite.

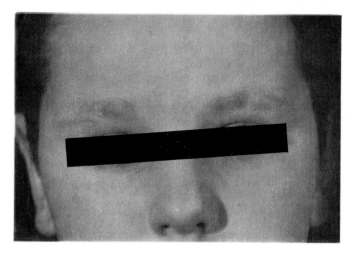

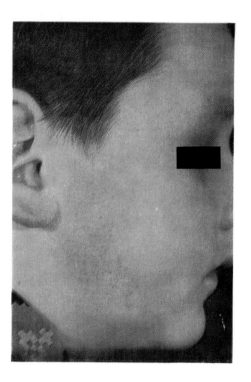

14 Ulerythema ophryogenes (UNNA and TAENZER)
Erythema, scaling, hair loss, and small follicular
hyperkeratoses of the eyebrows.

15 Ulerythema ophryogenes →
Persistent reticulated erythema with small follicular
horny papules (keratosis pilaris) extending to the cheeks.

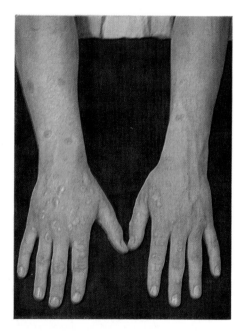

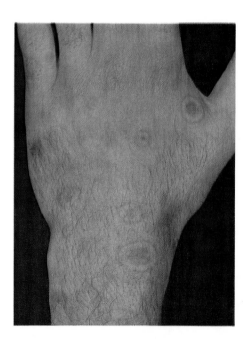

16 Erythema multiforme (VON HEBRA)
Early round, erythematous macules on
the extensor surface of the forearms
have subsequently developed raised,
pale borders and bluish-red centers.
These lesions (erythema iris) resemble
a cockade.

17 Erythema multiforme
Typical target lesions, formed by a new
crop of annular lesions. The older central macules show a darker red color;
the new peripheral lesions are pinkish.

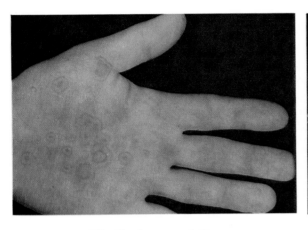

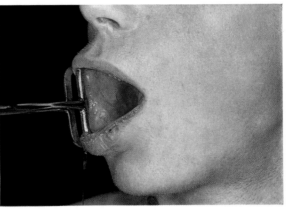

18   Erythema multiforme

In the same patient, several circinate lesions on the palm (inverse type) coalesce to form a gyrate pattern.

19   Erythema multiforme

Exudative erythematous lesions of the oral mucosa characteristic of the idiopathic type.

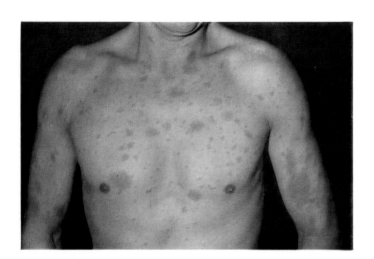

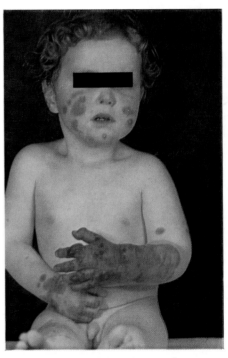

20   Erythema multiforme

Erythematous and papulovesicular patches in exanthematous distribution on the trunk.

21   Bullous erythema multiforme with hemorrhagic lesions   (drug eruption)

Rapid improvement following elimination of causative agent.

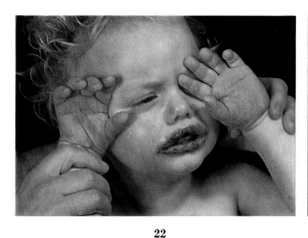
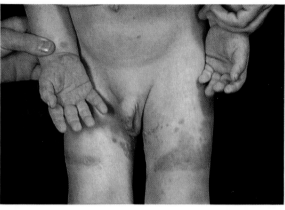

22 **23**

22 and 23   Stevens-Johnson syndrome
Bullous lesions, severe involvement of mucous membranes, conjunctivitis, malaise.

27   Erythema nodosum (von Hebra) →
Tender subcutaneous nodules with diffuse bright red
to violaceous erythema of overlying skin.

28   Erythema nodosum
Acute, painful, bright red, diffuse erythematous lesions
with subcutaneous edematous plaques and nodules.

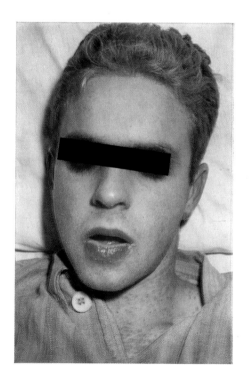
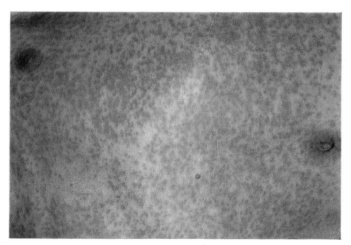

24 **25**

24, 25 and 26   Stevens-Johnson syndrome
24, 25 and 26   Stevens-Johnson syndrome. Macular, erythematous, edematous, and hemorrhagic lesions
in exanthematous distribution; involvement of mucous membranes.

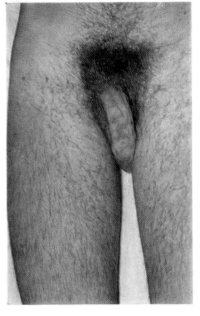

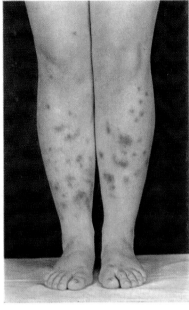

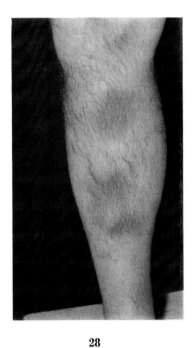

26   27   28

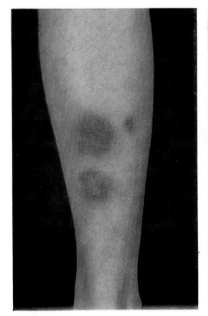

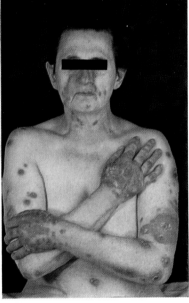

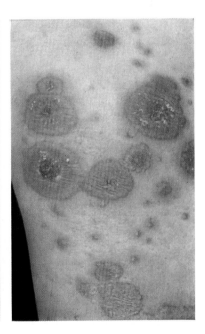

**29   Erythema nodosum, contusi-
form type**

Extravasation of blood into the subcutis causes a hematoma similar to that following a blunt injury (contusion).

30   Erythema elevatum diutinum
(Crocker and Williams)
Annular and oval, partially coalescing, slightly elevated nodules of varying size on the face and especially on the extensor aspects of the arms. Most lesions are reddish, those on the dorsa of the hands are brownish-red.

31   Erythema elevatum diutinum
Small new papules and nodules between large older annular plaques with central depression on the extensor aspects of the forearms.

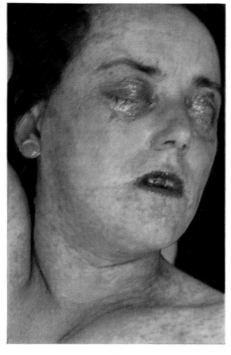

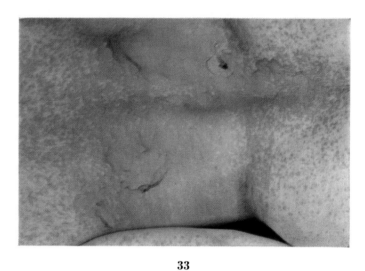

32   **33**

32 and 33   Toxic epidermal necrolysis (LYELL)

Extensive epidermolysis resembling scalding, with severe constitutional symptoms. Oral, tracheal, and vaginal mucous membranes as well as conjunctivae are involved. Probably drug eruption.

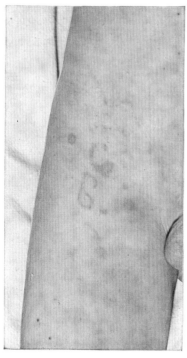

34   Erythema annulare rheumaticum
(LEHNDORF and LEINER)
Pale red to livid lesions in polycyclic configuration in a child with acute rheumatic fever.

35   Erythema annulare centrifugum (DARIER)
Annular and serpiginous erythematous lesions with raised urticarial border on the trunk.

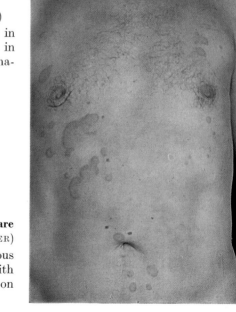

34   **35**

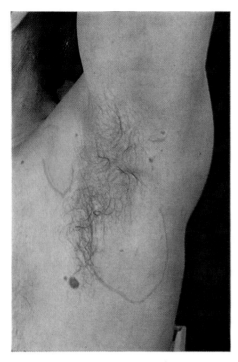

36 Erythema annulare centrifugum
(DARIER)

Gyrate macular lesions in the axillary
region. The urticarial component is less
pronounced.

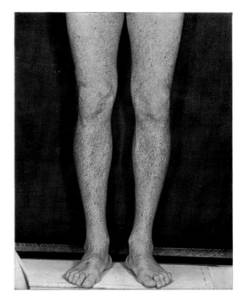

37 Hyperglobulinemic purpura
(WALDENSTRØM)

Multiple petechial lesions of the legs.

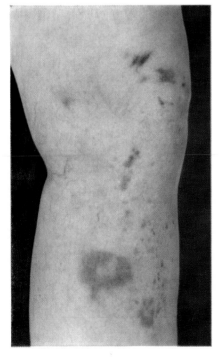

**38 Idiopathic thrombocytopenic
purpura** (WERLHOF)

Petechiae and ecchymoses.

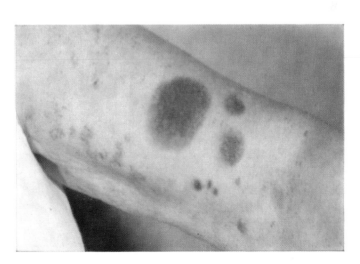

**39 Idiopathic thrombocytopenic
purpura** (WERLHOF)

Extensive ecchymoses.

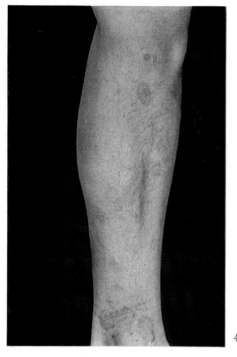
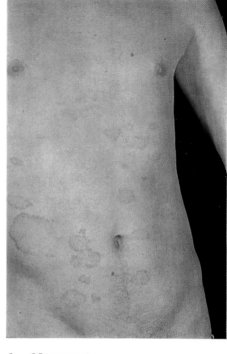

40   **41**

40 and **41**   **Purpura annularis telangiectodes** (MAJOCCHI)

Annular and polycyclic lesions with fine petechiae. Relatively early stage, evolving from small telangiectatic purpuric macules by centrifugal extension.

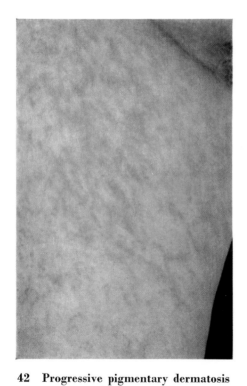

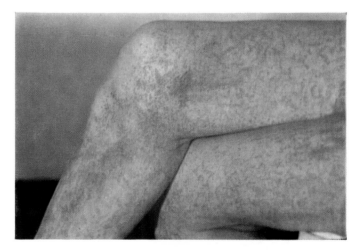

42   Progressive pigmentary dermatosis
(SCHAMBERG)

Large, partially coalescing, brownish-red macules of varying size and shape, with minute peripheral petechiae on the inner thigh.

43   Progressive pigmentary dermatosis
(SCHAMBERG)

Numerous petechiae on both legs.

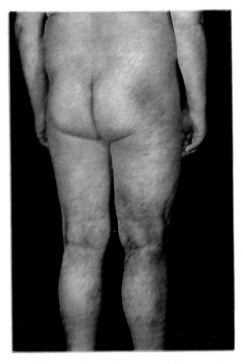

44   Progressive pigmentary dermatosis
(Schamberg)
Widespread involvement of legs and gluteal areas.

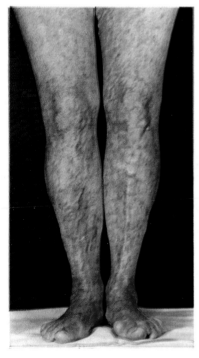

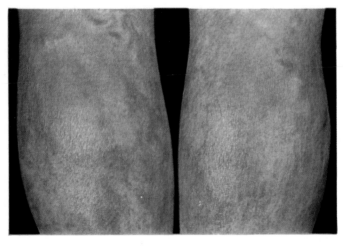

45   **46**

45 and 46   Pigmented purpuric lichenoid dermatitis (Gougerot-Blum)

The lesions resemble those of Schamberg's disease. In addition, they show densely grouped, flat, polygonal, lichenoid, pinhead-sized papules of brownish-red coloring resembling embedded grains of paprika.

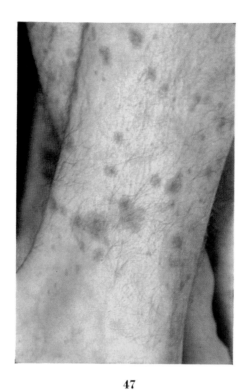

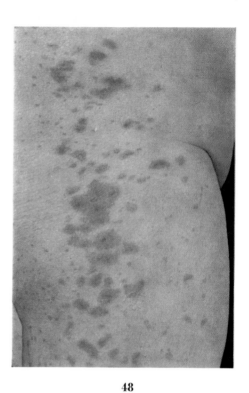

47   48

47 and **48   Schönlein's purpura**

Petechial hemorrhages of varying size, arranged symmetrically on the lower legs and thighs, particularly on extensor surfaces. On the thigh they appear as red macules with central hemorrhagic vesicles.

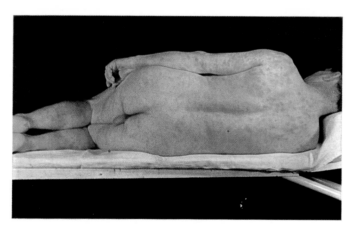

49   Purpura abdominalis (Schönlein-Henoch)

Widespread purpuric lesions associated with gastrointestinal symptoms.

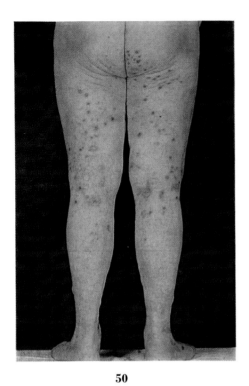

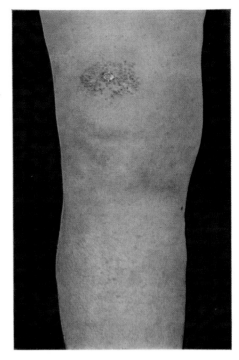

50   51

50 and **51**   **Triple syndrome of Gougerot**

Erythematous papular lesions in annular configuration, disseminated small petechiae, and cutaneous and subcutaneous nodules on the lower extremities.

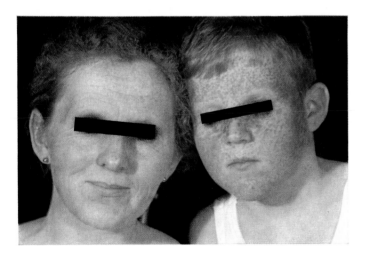

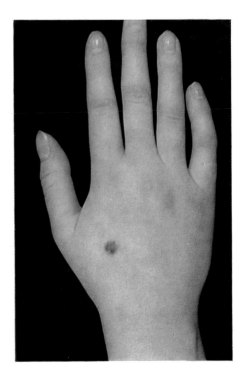

52   Freckles (ephelides)

Symmetrical, small hyperpigmented macules of exposed areas (mother and son).

53 Blue nevus (nevus caeruleus)

Sharply defined, small grayish-blue nodule.

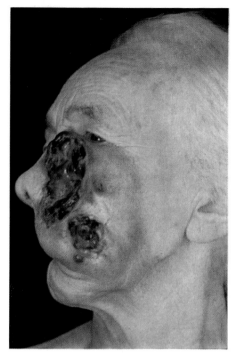

54 Melanosarcoma
Originating from a blue nevus. A very
rare complication.

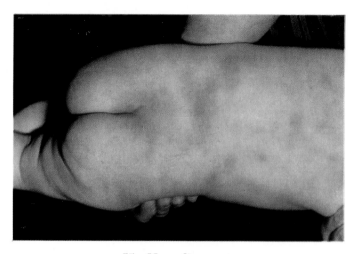

55 Mongolian spots
Diffuse grayish-blue discoloration in sacral region present
since birth.

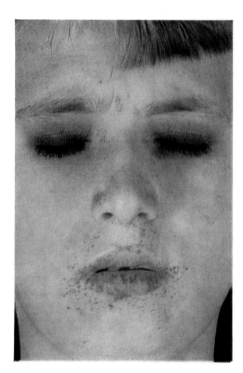

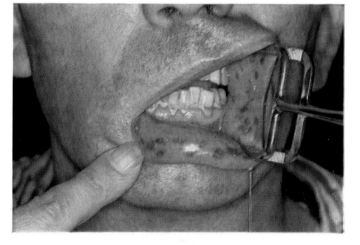

57 Pigmentation-polyposis syndrome
Pigmented spots of the oral mucosa
in a young adult.

56 Pigmentation-polyposis syndrome (Peutz-Jeghers). Numerous pigmented spots on the lips and about
the mouth. Oral mucosa not involved. Intestinal polyposis could not be demonstrated with certainty.
One sister and one brother of the patient showed similar perioral pigmentation. The mother of this 13-
year-old boy had died of malignant degeneration of intestinal polyposis.

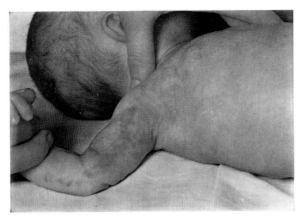 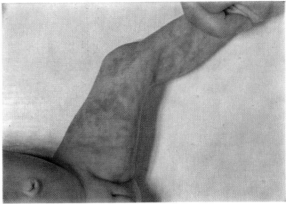

58   **59**

58 and **59**   **Incontinentia pigmenti** (Bloch-Sulzberger)
Bizarre, gyrate and band-like, grayish-brown pigmentation. Residual erythema still visible.

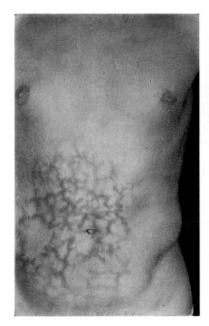 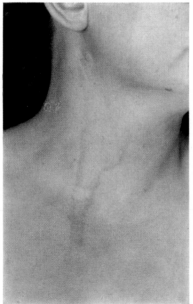 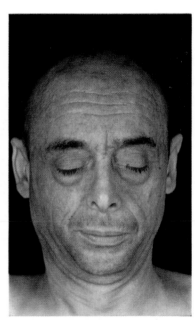

60   Melanodermia reticularis calorica

Reticular hyperpigmentation due to application of hot compresses.

61   Berloque dermatitis

Due to application of eau de cologne to the lateral areas of the neck, followed by sun exposure.

62   Riehl's melanosis

Diffuse hyperpigmentation of the face and neck.

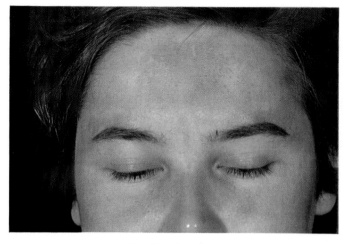

63 Vaselinoderma

Mottled hyperpigmentation of the forehead, ending abruptly
at the hairline, above which Vaseline was not applied.
Modern cosmetics rarely cause hyperpigmentation.

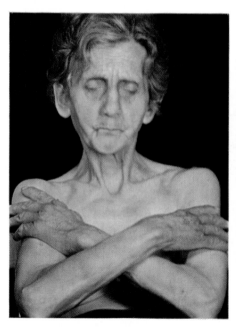

64 Pellagra

Brownish-red, sharply circumscribed
erythema involving areas exposed to
light, such as the face, neck, dorsa of
the hands, and wrists. Fine scaling of
the right hand.

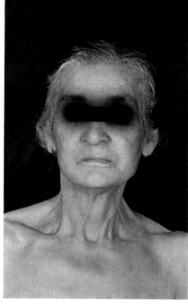

65 Pellagra

Sharply defined, scaling
livid erythema of the face,
neck, and nape of the neck
following a starvation diet.

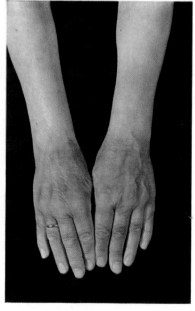

66 Pellagra

Brownish to livid erythema in
areas exposed to light. Associated with mental depression
and paresthesias.

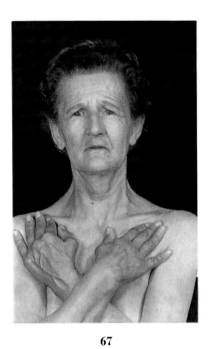

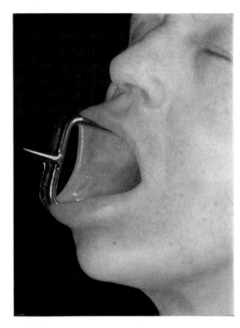

67

68

67 and **68**   **Addison's disease**

Typical, diffuse, brownish hyperpigmentation of the skin, and dark gray discoloration of the buccal mucosa.

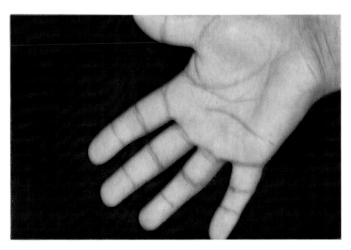

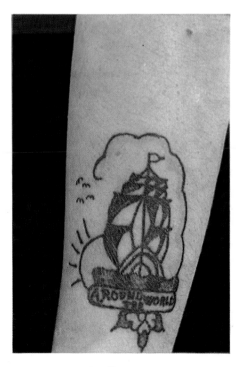

69   Addison's disease

Typical hyperpigmentation of the palmar creases.

70   Tattoo

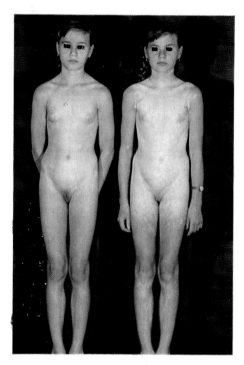

71   Vitiligo in twins

Widespread hypopigmentation of the trunk with sharply circumscribed
convex margin and slightly hyperpigmented border on the upper arms.

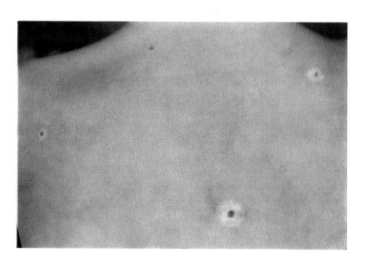

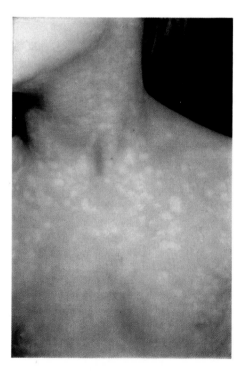

72   Sutton's perinevoid vitiligo (halo nevus)

Circular hypopigmentation around pigmented nevus.

73   Pseudoleukoderma

Following treatment of psoriasis with
ointments and ultraviolet irradiation.

Erythrodermas

A number of dermatoses associated with erythema and scaling and involving large areas of the integument are lumped together as exfoliative dermatoses or erythrodermas; their etiology is generally unknown. Common features of primary and secondary erythrodermas are diffuse redness associated with various types of scaling, elevated temperatures, chills, and pruritus.

Primary erythrodermas are those arising in normal skin (erythroderma associated with lymphomas, Hodgkin's disease, mycosis fungoides, etc.); *secondary erythrodermas* are seen when lesions of extensive dermatoses (chronic dermatitis, neurodermatitis, seborrheic eczema, psoriasis) spread to involve the entire body surface.

26

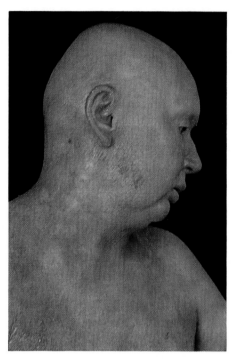

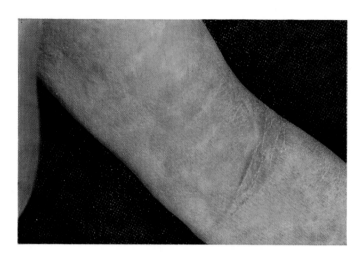

75 Primary erythroderma
In chronic myeloid leukemia. Mottled erythema, infiltration, and scaling.

74 Primary erythroderma
In chronic lymphatic leukemia. Dusky red erythema and scaling (l'homme rouge).

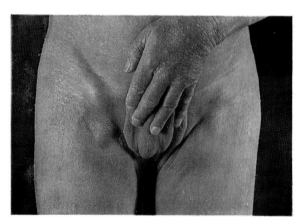

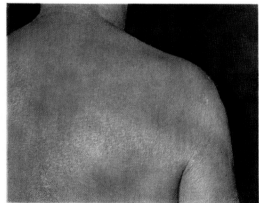

76 Primary erythroderma
Associated with lymphoma of the skin and lipomelanotic reticulosis of lymph nodes (PAUTRIER-WORINGER).

77 Primary erythroderma
In mycosis fungoides. Erythema, infiltration, fine scaling.

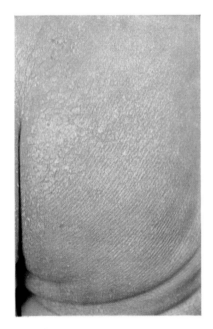

78   Secondary erythroderma

In psoriasis. Generalized erythema, whitish scaling, chills.

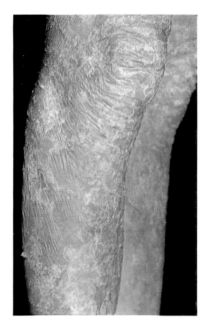

79   Secondary erythroderma

In psoriasis. Generalized erythema with characteristic large, silvery psoriatic scales.

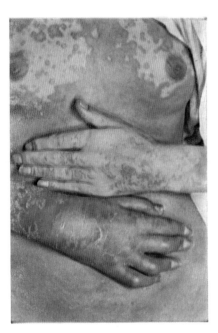

80   Secondary erythroderma

Islands of normal skin in psoriatic erythroderma.

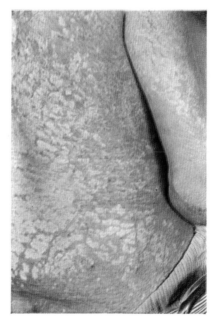

81   Secondary erythroderma

Some areas still show typical psoriatic silvery scales.

Papulosquamous eruptions

(Erythematosquamous diseases)

Psoriasis vulgaris

The sharply circumscribed lesions of psoriasis are covered with typical dry, silvery white, shiny micaceous scales. The erythemato-papulosquamous plaques arise from small, round, flat-topped, salmon-red papules, which are soon covered with thick white scales.

Diagnostic features are the "candle phenomenon" (scrapings of psoriatic scales resemble scrapings of a candle) and Auspitz's sign (minute bleeding points corresponding to the apices of the papillae are seen upon removal of the scales and a last thin epidermal membrane). Predilection sites are the elbows and knees (mechanical irritation) as well as the scalp and lumbosacral area, but other parts of the integument may be involved as well. According to site and configuration of the lesions, clinical differentiation is made between follicular, punctate, guttate, nummular, annular, gyrate, serpiginous, or confluent psoriasis. In acute stages of the disease, typical psoriatic lesions may develop in areas irritated by scratching or other nonspecific irritants (often in linear arrangement). This is called Koebner's phenomenon; it is not specific for psoriasis only. Special types of psoriasis are seen in certain skin regions.

Intertriginous psoriasis is found mostly in irritated areas of axillae and groins. *Hair growth* usually is not inhibited by the psoriatic process. *Fingernails* and *toenails* may show characteristic changes, particularly stippling of the nail plate, brownish or whitish discoloration, accumulation of scale on the nail bed, and separation of the distal portion of the nail plate. Psoriasis of the *palms* and *soles* may present diagnostic difficulties if no other skin areas are in involved. As in psoriatic changes of the nails, confusion with fungus infections must be avoided.

Pustular psoriasis is a rare clinical expression of the disease, characterized by the prevalence of microabscesses. Pustular psoriasis may be associated with chills, fever, arthritic pains, and a tendency to erythroderma (Zum-busch type). The Königsbeck-Barber-Ingram type, without systemic impairment, is usually limited to the distal extremities; it shows symmetrically arranged, grouped (but not confluent) pustules on red, scaly areas of the palms and soles, with psoriatic nail changes.

Occasionally, psoriasis may involve the small and large joints, particularly the distal phalanges of the fingers. Recurrent attacks may produce deformity and ankylosis of the joints. *Arthropathic psoriasis* is often difficult to differentiate from other degenerative processes of the joints. Suggestive features are involvement of distal joints, typical x-ray findings and absence of rheumatoid factors in the serum.

The etiology and pathogenesis of psoriasis are not clear. A positive family history can be obtained in many patients.

Acrodermatitis continua suppurativa (Hallopeau)

This disease may be related to psoriasis. It is often preceded by trauma. After initial paronychial changes of the fingers or toes, continuous crops of coalescent pustules appear, lifting the epidermis and forming lakes of pus. The process terminates in atrophy of the skin and loss of the nails. Involvement of the palms and soles is not uncommon. Occasionally, generalization may occur, making differentiation from pustular psoriasis extremely difficult. A bacterial etiology cannot be ruled out in some patients.

Acrodermatitis enteropathica (Danbold-Closs)

The classification of this disorder is difficult. It is a disease of early childhood and often ends fatally. Rarely, it may occur in young adults who have a typical history of exacerbations and remissions since childhood. Squamous, erythemato-vesiculo-bullous skin changes near body orifices and on the acra are accompanied by diffuse alopecia, chronic paronychia, partial or total loss of nails, diarrhea, and photophobia. Recent reports suggest that it is a hereditary disease. Good response to treatment with diiodohydroxyquinoline and iodochlorhydroxyquin has been used as a diagnostic criterion.

Parapsoriasis

The parapsoriasis group has no direct relationship to psoriasis. It includes three rare varieties of widespread scaling eruptions on the trunk and extremities. Their etiology is unknown; they are notoriously resistant to treatment and follow a chronic course.

Lichenoid parapsoriasis
(Pityriasis lichenoides chronica [JULIUSBERG])

New, small, red, round lichenoid lesions covered with fine scales develop next to older, paler, flat-topped lesions, each of which is covered with a grayish-white, thick scale. Most lesions persist indefinitely. In some cases, a leukoderma remains after complete involution of the eruption.

Parapsoriasis en plaques
(Erythrodermie pityriasique en plaques disseminées [BROCQ])

This chronic disorder causes no discomfort. It is characterized by circumscribed yellowish to reddish-brown pseudoatrophic macular lesions with a very fine adherent scale. The plaques, which may reach the size of a hand, occur on trunk and extremities. Differential diagnosis includes mycosis fungoides, which may have a similar onset. Increasing infiltration and pruritus are distinguishing features.

Retiform parapsoriasis
(Parakeratosis variegata [UNNA])

Yellowish-red, flat-topped scaling papules become confluent in an annular or retiform pattern. Late changes are atrophy, pigmentary disturbances, and telangiectasias. Transition to mycosis fungoides has been observed.

Varioliform parapsoriasis
(Pityriasis lichenoides et varioliformis acuta [MUCHA-HABERMANN])

In contrast to chronic forms of parapsoriasis, this disorder is probably due to primary vascular changes. It is now classified as an acute form of necrotizing vasculitis of unknown etiology. Following febrile infections, exanthematous eruptions appear with papulovesicular and hemorrhagic or necrotic lesions which often leave varioliform scars.

Pityriasis rosea (GIBERT)

A relatively large, pink to fawn primary lesion ("herald patch"), usually located on the trunk, is followed by small, pityriasiform, faintly scaling, slightly erythematous, round to oval patches showing a typical crinkly scale ("collarette") at the border. These secondary lesions are arranged in an exanthematous symmetrical pattern; their long axes run parallel to the lines of cleavage of the skin. They tend to heal spontaneously after several weeks, leaving immunity. The etiology of the disease is unknown, although many factors suggest an infectious origin.

Pityriasis rubra pilaris (DEVERGIE)

This rare chronic dermatosis, which may occur in any age group, is characterized by disseminated erythematosquamous salmon-pink to reddish-brown plaques, with yellow to black, perifollicular, acuminate horny plugs (often pierced by a hairshaft), which produce a rough, grater-like surface. The areas frequently involved are the extensor aspects of the extremities, dorsa of hands and fingers, flexor aspects of the joints, chest, face, neck, and abdomen. Generalized involvement, leaving characteristic irregular islands of skin intact, and transition to an exfoliative dermatitis are not uncommon. Palms and soles often are covered with fissured thick hyperkeratotic scaling masses (keratodermic sandal). The scalp may show severe pityriasiform scaling. Grayish-white patches of the oral mucosa, resembling the lesions of lichen planus, are rare. Instances suggesting a hereditary factor in the etiology of the disease have been reported.

Lichen planus

Predilection sites of this disease are the flexor aspects of the upper extremities, the lateral aspects of the trunk, and the penis; the lips, the mucous membranes of the mouth (tongue), and (rarely) the face also may be involved. The typical lesions, confined to the natural lines of the skin, are small, salmon-colored to bluish-lavender, polygonal, flat-topped papules with a smooth, shiny surface; they grow in number to form large patches and are usually associated with slight scaling and varying degrees of pruritus. In acute exanthematous exacerbations with more pronounced inflammation, the primary lesions have a more circular shape. Diascopy of the larger lesions with a glass slide reveals a lacy network of white streaks (WICKHAM's striae). New lesions often appear in linear fashion along scratch marks (KOEBNER phenomenon). The following clinical variations of the disease are common.

Lichen planus annularis atrophicans is characterized by annular arrangement of lesions retaining the papular margin while the center becomes atrophic. Semicircular arrangement results in a picture resembling tuberoserpiginous syphilitic plaques.

Other variants show thick hyperkeratotic lesions (*lichen planus verrucosus*) on the anterior aspect of the lower legs and on the scrotum, or transformation of flat-topped nodules into pointed lesions *(lichen planus acuminatus)*. *Lichen planus pemphigoides* is characterized by the formation of bullae, which are usually surrounded by more typical lesions.

Involvement of mucous membranes, particularly of the buccal mucosa, may be seen in addition to or without skin changes. These lesions have a distinctive linear white lacy pattern. On the tongue, they may simulate leukoplakia; on the lips, they have the appearance of a drop of paraffin. The cause of the disease is not known.

A special follicular form of lichen planus is *lichen planopilaris* (LASSUEUR-GRAHAM-LITTLE syndrome) with cicatricial alopecia of the scalp.

Many cases of pseudopelade of BROCQ are probably related to this type of lichen planus.

Lichen nitidus (PINKUS)

Lichen nitidus is probably not related to lichen planus. Pinhead-sized, discrete, skin-colored or reddish-brown, shiny, flat-topped papules covered with small scales appear, sometimes in patches, on the shaft of the penis, the flexor surfaces of the wrists and forearms (occasionally in linear arrangement), and, rarely, in other body areas (axillae, palms). The lesions itch only slightly and show no tendency toward growth or confluence. Instances of high familial incidence have been observed. Diagnosis is based on histological examination. The lesions may remain unchanged for many years.

Acanthosis nigricans

This dermatosis does not belong to the group of papulosquamous eruptions; it is not related to other skin diseases.

Symmetrically arranged, sharply defined, flesh-colored to brownish papules occur on the neck, corners of mouth, axillae, umbilical area, external genitals and chest. The skin markings become intensified; their surface later becomes deeply furrowed and verrucous. Eventually, the lesions develop into irregular, hyperpigmented grayish to black patches of velvety papillary hypertrophy. The cause of this skin affection is unknown. Three forms may be distinguished.

The *malignant type* has about the same incidence in both sexes, and usually manifests itself in middle or late life.

It is rapidly progressive, often associated with pruritus, and has no typical sites of predilection. Endocrine disturbances are absent. The role of hereditary factors is not clear. Hyperpigmentation is pronounced. This type is associated with a high incidence of internal cancer, particularly abdominal adenocarcinomas. The skin lesions themselves never become malignant.

The *benign type* is a genodermatosis, probably related to endocrine changes during puberty. The disease predominantly affects the female sex, usually manifests itself in early childhood or at puberty, is rarely associated with pruritus, and has a high familial incidence. It may remain stationary or show spontaneous regression.

A third type, *pseudoacanthosis nigricans*, occurs in obese patients, usually before puberty, but may also start later. Endocrine disturbances associated with obesity, such as diabetes, thyroid dysfunction, or CUSHING's syndrome, may be observed simultaneously. The skin changes show no progressive tendency, the lesions are less markedly pigmented. Predilection sites are axillae, neck and anogenital region.

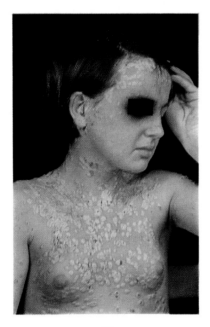

82

82, 83 and 84   Psoriasis

Widespread, sharply circumscribed, discrete and coalescent patches with typical dry, silvery white thick scales; also early, small, salmon-red scaling papules.

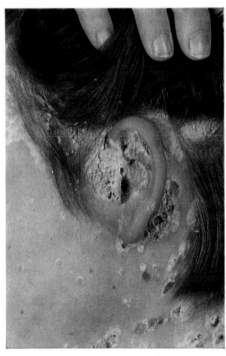

83

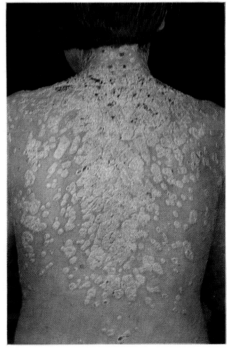

84

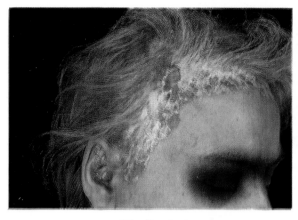

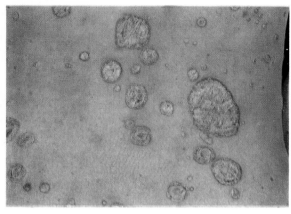

85 Psoriasis

Sharply marginated lesions of the scalp, forehead, and ears with thick white scales.

86 Psoriasis

Punctate, guttate, and nummular lesions of the back.

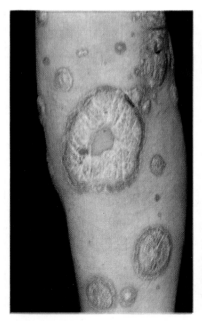

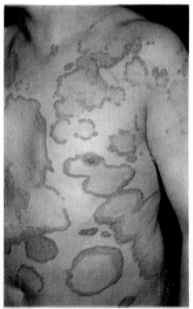

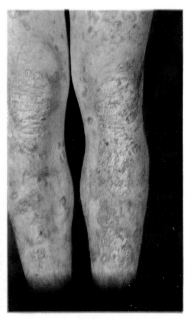

87 Psoriasis

Annular psoriasis of the leg with heavy scaling and clear center.

88 Psoriasis

Figurate psoriasis of the trunk with active border and clear, slightly hyperpigmented center.

89 Psoriasis

Typical areas of predilection on extensor surfaces of the legs, particularly on the knees.

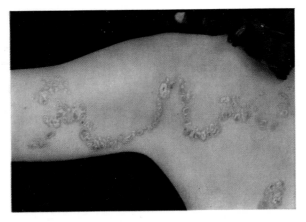

90　Psoriasis
Gyrate psoriasis, resembling tuberoserpiginous syphilid.

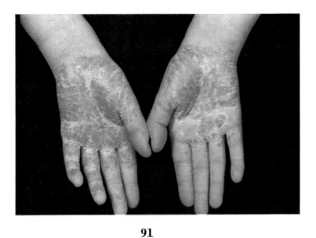

91

91 and **92　Psoriasis of palms and soles**
Sharply marginated erythema with lamellar
exfoliation.

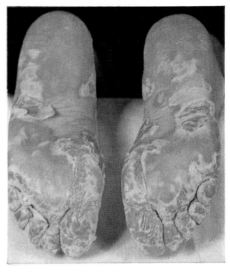

92

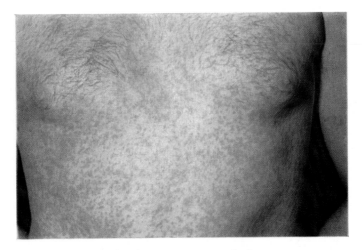

93　Acute guttate psoriasis
Immediately following a generalized drug eruption, psoriatic lesions appeared in the same
areas in a patient with a tendency to psoriasis (Koebner phenomenon).

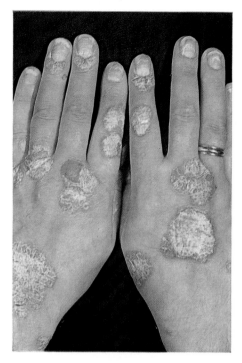

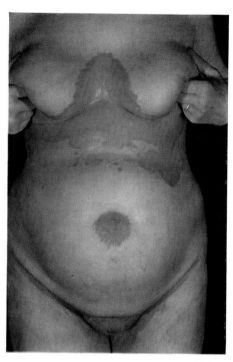

94   Psoriasis of the hands
Typical nummular patches with involvement of nail folds and secondary nail changes.

95   Intertriginous psoriasis
Differentiation from seborrheic eczema may be difficult.

96 and 97   Psoriatic fingernails
Brownish (oily) discoloration and punctate stippling of the nail plate.

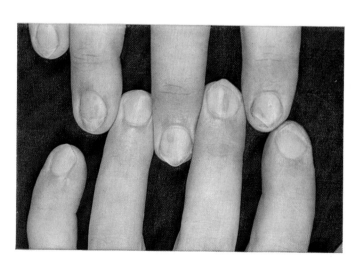

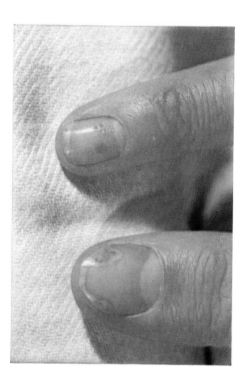

96

97

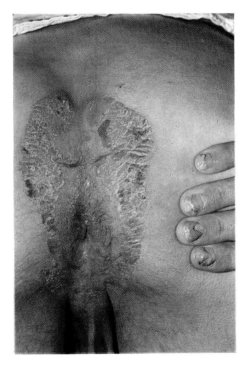

98 Psoriasis of the anal region and of the fingernails

Sharply marginated lesions.

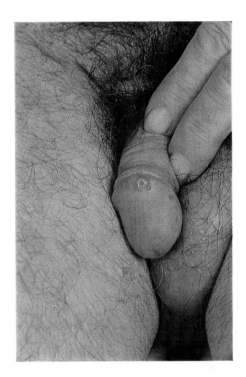

99 Psoriasis of the glans penis

Isolated round erythematosquamous lesions.

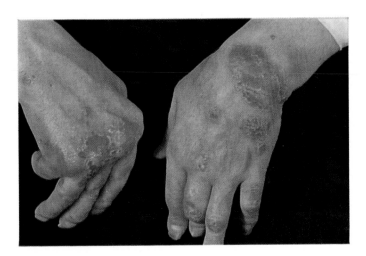

100 Arthropathic psoriasis

Deformity and ankylosis of the small joints, associated with typical skin lesions.

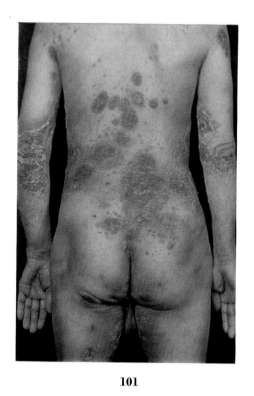

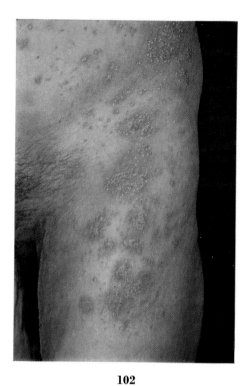

101

102

101 and **102**   **Psoriasis; pustular type** (VON ZUMBUSCH)

Erythematosquamous patches studded with many small pustules. Severe constitutional symptoms.

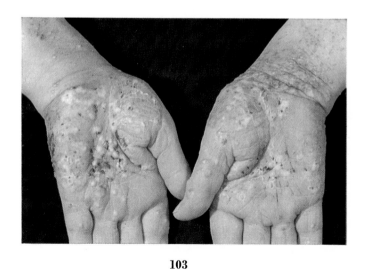

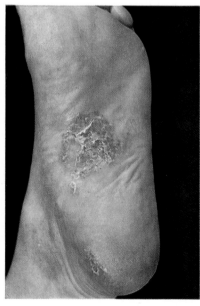

103

103 and **104**   **Psoriasis; pustular type** (BARBER)

Pustular eruption of the hands and feet. No systemic changes.

104

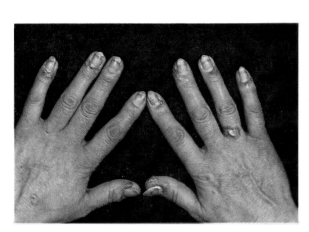

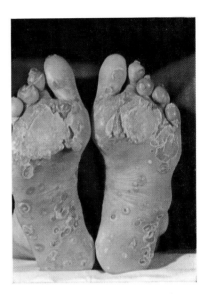

105

106

105 and **106**   **Acrodermatitis continua suppurativa** (HALLOPEAU)
Inflammatory changes of nail folds, finger tips, toes, and soles.

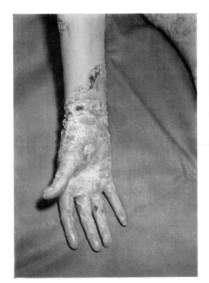

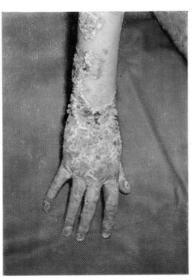

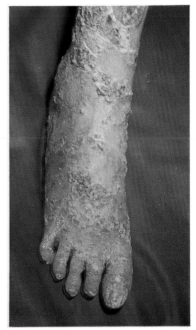

107

108

107, 108 and **109**   **Acrodermatitis continua suppurativa** (HALLOPEAU)
Severe type with tendency toward generalization. Lakes of pus and
thick yellowish crusts. Tips of fingers smooth and atrophic.

109

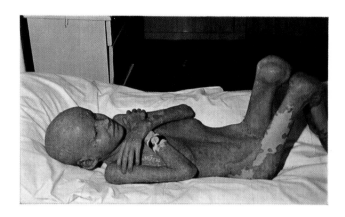

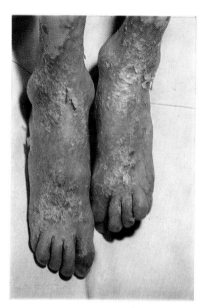

110

111

110 and **111**   **Acrodermatitis enteropathica** (Danbolt-Closs)

Advanced cachectic stage with contractures. Erythroderma with marked scaling and pustular lesions; total alopecia, loss of nails. Blepharitis and photophobia.

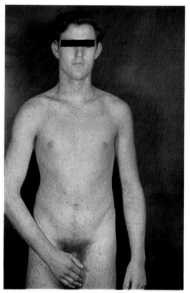

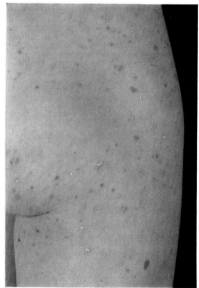

112   Lichenoid parapsoriasis (pityriasis lichenoides chronica Juliusberg). Numerous persistent small red lichenoid lesions covered with fine scales.

113   Lichenoid parapsoriasis (pityriasis lichenoides chronica Juliusberg). Fresh, erythematous lichenoid lesions beside older lesions which are less erythematous and show typical flat-topped papules with grayish-white thick scales.

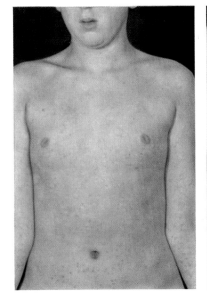

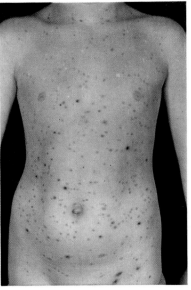

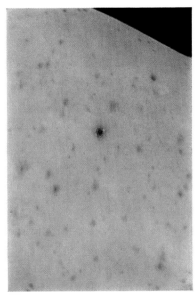

114 Lichenoid parapsoriasis (pityriasis lichenoides chronica Juliusberg)

Subsiding papular and erythematous eruption of chest and arms.

115 Acute varioliform parapsoriasis (pityriasis lichenoides et varioliformis acuta Mucha-Habermann)

Papulovesicular hemorrhagic and necrotic lesions in exanthematous distribution.

116 Acute varioliform parapsoriasis (pityriasis lichenoides et varioliformis acuta Mucha-Habermann)

Discrete papules, vesicles, and necrotic lesions on upper back.

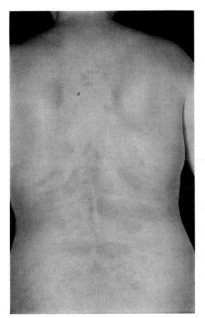

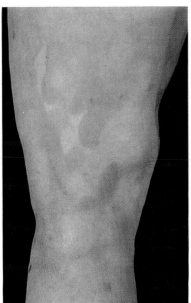

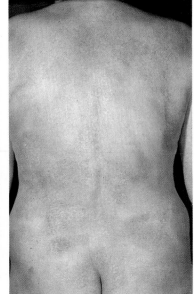

117 **118**

119 Mycosis fungoides

117 and 118 Parapsoriasis en plaques (erythrodermie pityriasique en plaques disseminées Brocq)

Brownish-red, round, bandlike plaques and irregularly outlined, pityriasiform, pseudoatrophic lesions. No infiltration, no pruritus.

In contrast to parapsoriasis en plaques (which may precede mycosis fungoides) the lesions are pruritic and more infiltrated.

40

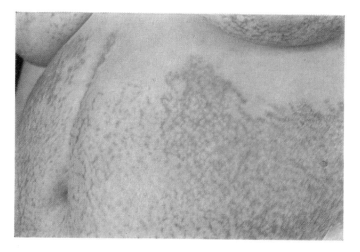

120   Retiform parapsoriasis (parakeratosis variegata Unna)
Yellowish-red, flat-topped scaling papules in annular and
retiform arrangement with telangiectatic, atrophic, and pigmentary changes.

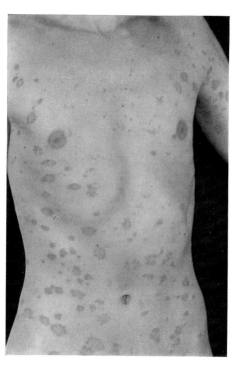

121   Pityriasis rosea
Disseminated eruption of salmon-red,
oval, maculopapular lesions with pityriasiform fine scaling.

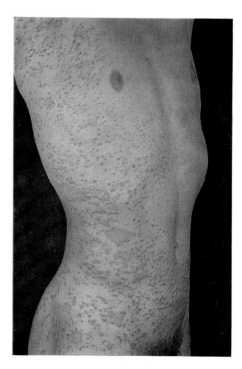

122   Pityriasis rosea
Aggravated by topical treatment. Distribution of lesions following lines of
cleavage of the skin.

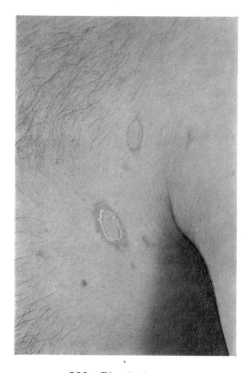

123   Pityriasis rosea
Primary plaque (herald patch) and secondary lesions, showing a typical thin,
crinkly scale (collarette) at the border.

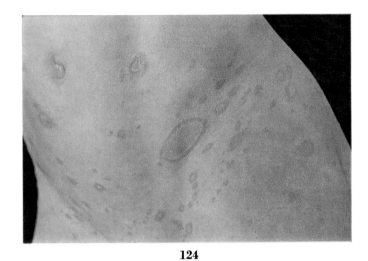

124   Pityriasis rosea
Primary plaque and secondary
lesions. Typical marginal scaling
(collarette).

124

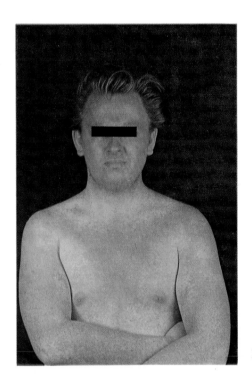

125

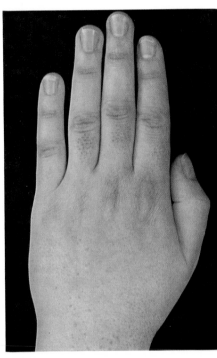

126

125, 126 and **127   Pityriasis rubra pilaris**
(DEVERGIE)
Discrete pinhead-sized follicular papules with central horny plugs in symmetrical distribution, surrounded by islands of normal skin. Dorsa of fingers
and hands are frequently involved;
they show a typical "nutmeg grater"
surface.

127

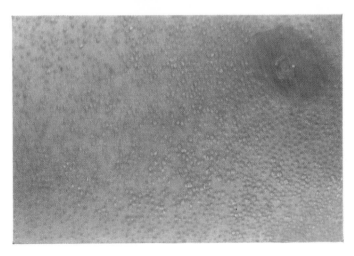

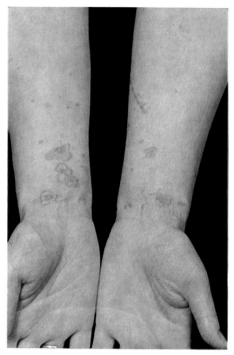

128   Lichen planus

Typical involvement of the wrists; salmon-colored to bluish-red, polygonal, flat-topped pruritic papules with a smooth shiny surface. Linear Koebner phenomenon on the ulnar aspect of the left forearm.

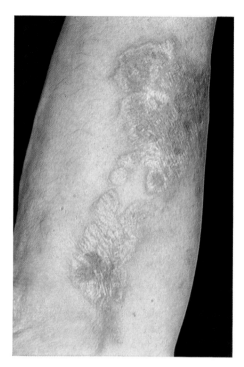

129   Annular lichen planus

A rare variant of lichen planus. Characteristic bluish-red color; marked pruritus.

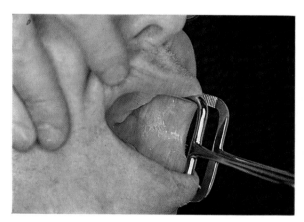

130   Lichen planus of oral mucosa

Distinctive linear and reticulate white lacy pattern.

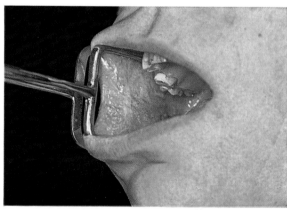

131   Lichen planus of lips and oral mucosa

Typical white discoloration of buccal mucous membrane.

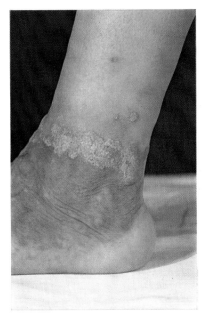

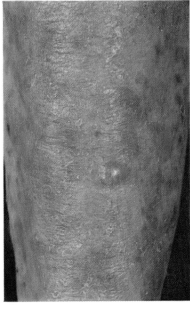

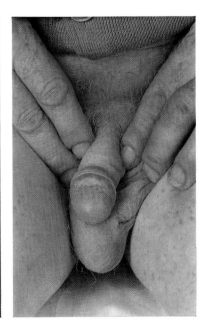

132 Hypertrophic lichen planus
Elevated pruritic verrucous plaque on the lower leg.

133 Bullous lichen planus
Large bulla surrounded by typical lichen planus lesions.

134 Lichen planus of the glans penis
Frequent location of lichen planus

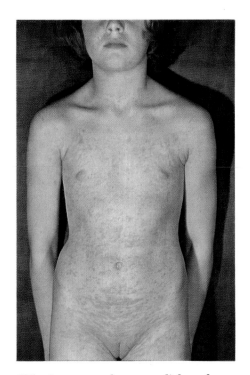

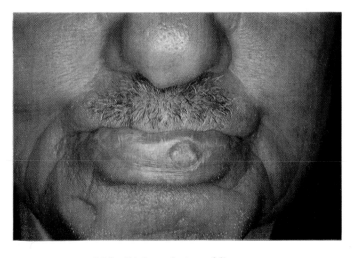

136 Lichen planus of lips
Associated with squamous cell cancer, a rare complication.

135 Acute exanthematous lichen planus
Symmetrical lichenoid lesions; often non-pruritic.

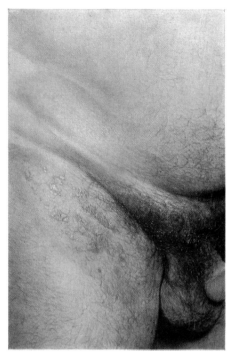

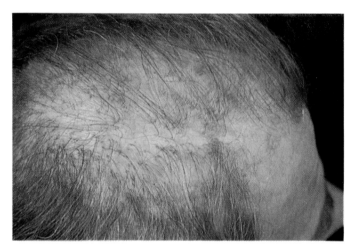

137 Lichen planus superimposed on circumscribed scleroderma

A very rare combination.

138 Lichen planopilaris (Graham-Little syndrome)

Cicatricial alopecia of the scalp with follicular lesions of lichen planus.

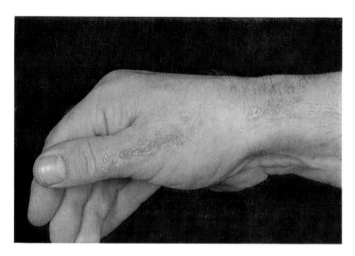

139 Lichen planopilaris (Graham-Little syndrome)

Typical lichen planus lesions of the hand in same patient as in figure 138.

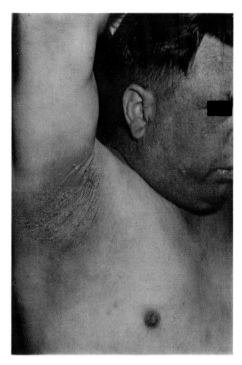

140   Acanthosis nigricans

Marked hyperpigmentation of axillae,
face, and neck with hypertrophic axillary folds, characteristic of malignant
type. No tumor has been found yet in
this patient.

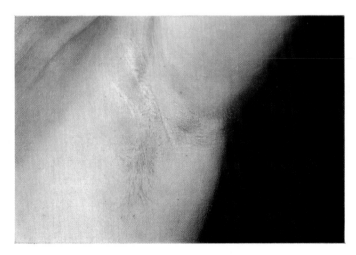

141   Acanthosis nigricans, benign form

Usually seen in young female patients with endocrine disturbances. High familial incidence.

Dermatitis-Eczema Group

Dermatitis-eczema

The terms dermatitis and eczema are used for a characteristic sequence of inflammatory changes of the epidermis and upper dermis which can be induced by a variety of irritants, allergens and other factors. In the past, the term eczema was used for different chronic forms of dermatitis. In modern usage, it is meaningless without qualifying adjectives and should best be avoided.

The characteristic sequence of dermatitic skin changes consists mainly of erythematous and edematous patches, followed by papules, vesicles, and oozing. Mild to severe pruritus is usually present. Scaling, erosions, crusts, and circumscribed lichenification are seen in later stages of the disease.

Contact dermatitis

Skin changes in contact dermatitis start in areas of contact with the irritating or allergenic agent. The reaction is usually localized and limited to the area of exposure. Two main types of contact dermatitis can be differentiated. *Primary irritant (toxic) contact dermatitis* may occur in any individual, without prior exposure, shortly after contact with an offending substance of sufficient strength. *Allergic contact dermatitis* occurs only in sensitized individuals. Repeated exposure to the same agent is necessary to induce dermatitic changes which appear after an incubation period of varying length. Once the patient is sensitized, even minimal contact may cause exacerbation. *Id reactions*, possibly due to autosensitization, can be seen in severe cases of contact dermatitis in regions distant from the original contact area, often in widespread distribution.

Common contact allergens and diagnostic methods are described in the discussion of Cutaneous Allergy.

Nummular dermatitis

This common clinical variety of the dermatitis-eczema group is characterized by pruritic, coin-like (nummular), oozing patches, frequently located on the extensor surfaces of arms, hands, and legs. Sometimes it is related to an exacerbation of other chronic eczematous processes, particularly of the lower legs. In patients with an atopic history it is considered an exudative form of neurodermatitis (in contrast to the dry form, lichen simplex chronicus); in other patients it represents a clinically distinct form of contact dermatitis.

Seborrheic dermatitis (Unna)

Perifollicular, pinhead-sized, erythematous pink or yellowish lesions which grow into macular patches appear on the scalp and face, in the retroauricular, presternal, and interscapular areas, in the umbilical region, in the gluteal crease, axillae and genital area. The dermatitis is usually confined to areas richly supplied with sebaceous glands. Round or oval, polycyclic, and punctate perifollicular lesions may arise simultaneously or in succession. As the originally pinkish macules increase in size, they assume a yellowish coloring and are covered with greasy scales and dirty yellow crusts. Typical eczematous changes (papulovesicles, exudative lesions) are seen only occasionally, and then only in the marginal areas of the lesions. Increased sebum production and hyperhidrosis provide the basis for microbial action and inflammatory changes, which lead to sensitization and thus help maintain the dermatitis. A lowered resistance to superficial bacterial infection favors the formation and persistence of seborrheic dermatitis.

Atopic dermatitis (Coca-Sulzberger)
(Disseminated neurodermatitis Brocq)
(Prurigo diathesique Besnier)

Atopic dermatitis often starts in infancy, affecting the lateral aspects of the face; two-thirds of the cases of so-called "infantile eczema" are early manifestations of atopic dermatitis. There is usually a family or personal history of atopy, e.g., atopic dermatitis, urticaria, asthma, or hay fever.

The typical facial lesions are followed in childhood by eczematous eruptions involving the flexor surfaces of the arms and legs, the dorsa of the hands, and the wrists. Lichenification, the principal criterion of atopic dermatitis, is predominant. The disease reaches its maximum in extent and severity during the second and third decades, then gradually subsides. Each episode starts with violent attacks of pruritus, probably related to excessive dryness of the skin. These attacks, which particularly occur at nighttime, provoke furious scratching which promotes lichenification and secondary infection of the skin. The lichenified skin of the forehead, antecubital and popliteal fossae, the characteristic frustrated facial expression, the broken off lateral portions of the eyebrows (Hertogue's sign), and the atopic pleats of the eyelids are typical diagnostic features.

Not infrequently, ophthalmologic examination with a slit lamp reveals a cataract. The most serious, potentially fatal complication of atopic dermatitis is superinfection with herpes simplex or vaccina virus which has a tendency to become generalized. Both complications, *eczema herpeticum* and *eczema vaccinatum*, will be discussed in the chapter on virus infections of the skin.

Lichen simplex chronicus (Vidal)
(Circumscribed neurodermatitis Brocq)

This severely pruritic disorder is a separate form of neurodermatitis, easily distinguishable from the generalized (disseminated, diffuse) type. The striate lesions or solitary circumscribed round to ovoid lichenified patches are usually seen in middle aged patients, primarily on the inner aspects of the thighs, the extensor aspects of the lower legs, and in the occipital-nuchal region. The lichenified areas are the result of constant scratching and rubbing.

Prurigo nodularis (Hyde)

This rare disease is closely related to circumscribed neurodermatitis. Isolated dome-shaped, dark, itching nodules which may reach a diameter of 1 to 2 cm. occur on extremities, in the face, and occasionally on the trunk. The surrounding skin may be normal or lichenified. The nodules usually show an excoriated and verrucous surface.

Fox-Fordyce disease

This rare dermatosis does not belong to the dermatitis-eczema group. It occurs mostly in women, primarily involving the axillae, the mammillary and umbilical regions, the external genitals, and the inner aspects of the thighs, i.e., areas amply supplied with apocrine sweat glands. Characteristic features are discrete, small, firm, follicular, skin-colored or yellowish conical papules, tormenting pruritus, and exacerbation during menstruation. The hairs are broken off, whereas the surrounding skin is not appreciably changed. The skin markings are normal in contrast to circumscribed neurodermatitis. The disorder is considered a form of apocrine miliaria by many authors.

48

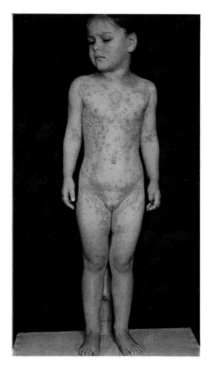

142   Seborrheic dermatitis
Typical localization of symmetrical follicular and macular
erythematosquamous lesions with greasy yellow scales.

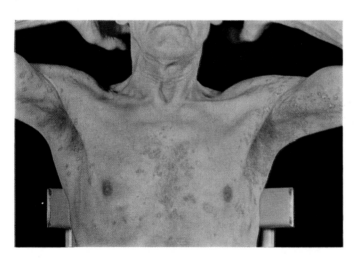

143   Seborrheic dermatitis
Typical involvement of sternal area and axillae.

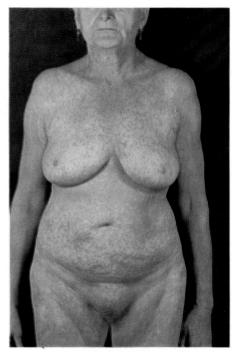

144   Seborrheic dermatitis
Coalescing follicular and macular lesions. Transition to seborrheic erythroderma.

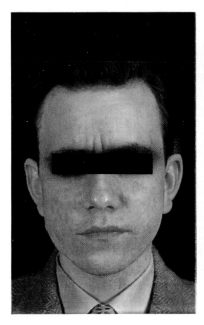

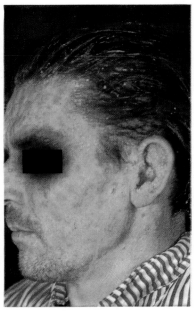

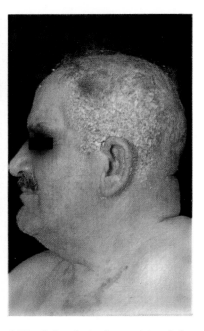

145   Seborrheic dermatitis of the face

Irregular erythema and mild scaling.

146   Seborrheic dermatitis of the face

Characteristic greasy yellowish scales of scalp and ears.

147   Seborrheic dermatitis of the scalp and face

Massive dry and greasy scaling of scalp.

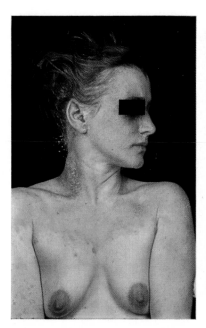

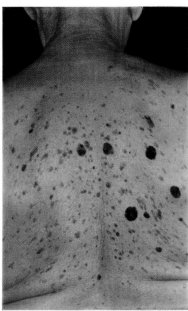

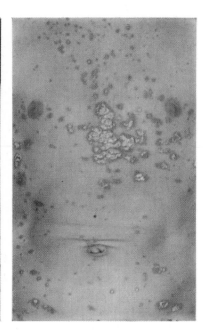

148   Seborrheic dermatitis

Involvement of scalp, ears, face, neck, and upper chest.

149   Seborrheic keratoses

Greasy, raised keratotic tumors (not related to seborrheic dermatitis).

150   Psoriasiform seborrheic dermatitis

Closely related to psoriasis (seborrhiasis).

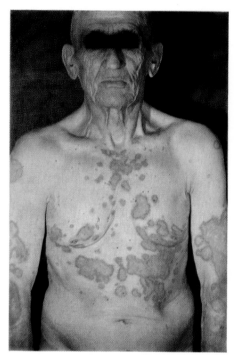

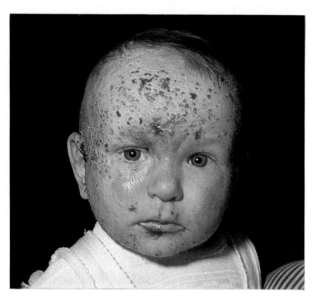

**151 Figurate seborrheic derma-
titis**

Sharply defined patches with
irregular border.

152 Seborrheic dermatitis in an infant

Erythematosquamous lesions of the face
associated with seborrheic cradle cap.

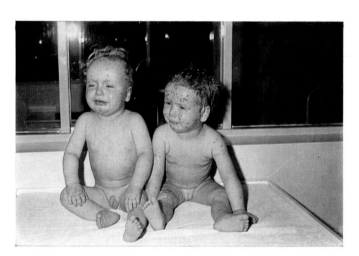

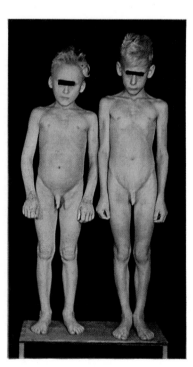

153 Atopic dermatitis in twins

Pruritic excoriated lesions of the face and extremities.

154 Atopic dermatitis in brothers

Dry lichenified eczematous eruption of the face and extremities.

154

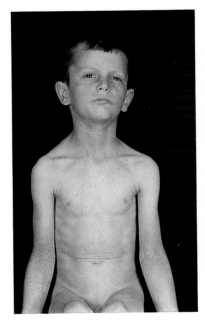

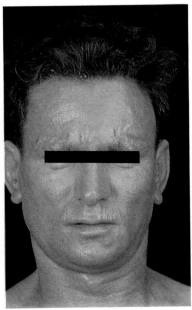

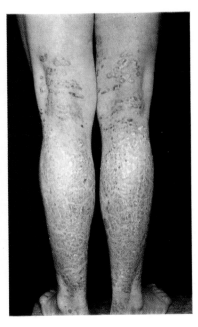

155   Atopic dermatitis
Flexural eczema of antecubital
areas of both arms.

156   Atopic dermatitis
Erythema, scaling, lichenification,
and loss of lateral portion of eyebrows due to rubbing and
scratching.

157   Lichen simplex chronicus
(VIDAL)
(Circumscribed neurodermatitis
BROCQ)
Thick, lichenified, pruritic lesions
of the legs.

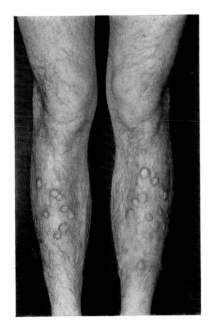

158   Prurigo nodularis (HYDE)
Dome-shaped pruritic nodules with verrucous surface.

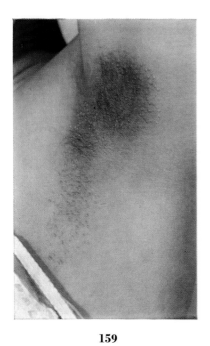

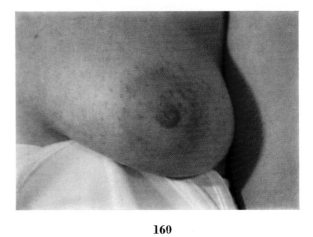

159

160

159 and **160**   **Fox-Fordyce disease**
Discrete, pruritic, conical follicular papules in the axillae and around the nipples.

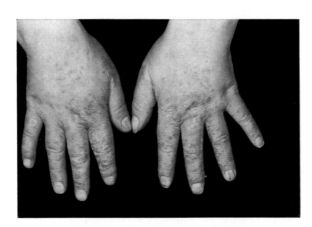

161   Chronic irritant dermatitis
Pruritic eczematous patches of the dorsa of the hands (housewife's eczema).

Cutaneous Allergy

Allergy is an acquired specific alteration in the capacity to react, brought about by interaction of an antigen with its specific antibody. Anaphylaxis, idiosyncrasy, hypersensitivity reaction are medical terms of historical importance; these responses are now classified as different types of allergic reaction. The concept of immunity has become somewhat separated from the more comprehensive concept of allergy; both are antigen-antibody mechanisms, respectively leading to pathogenic (allergy) and nonpathogenic (immunity) responses of the organism.

Antigens (allergens) are substances which induce the formation of specific proteins (antibodies). The ability of antigens to combine with their antibodies produces complex antigen-antibody reactions, which are the fundamental mechanism of *allergy*.

Two types of allergic reactions are recognized.

1. *Immediate reaction:* In the presence of serum antibodies, clinical symptoms appear within minutes after introduction of the specific antigen (e.g., serum sickness, bronchial asthma, urticaria, reactions to parasites, and some drug allergies). Circulating antibodies may be demonstrated with the PRAUSNITZ-KÜSTNER reaction.

2. *Delayed reaction:* Clinical symptoms manifest themselves after 12 to 48 hours (e.g., allergy of infection and allergic contact dermatitis).

Allergic cutaneous reactions

A number of substances may elicit allergic skin reactions, such as morbilliform, scarlatiniform, urticarial, hemorrhagic, erythema multiforme-like, and fixed drug eruptions (which consistently occur at the same site following oral or parenteral administration of the antigen).

Drug allergy

Virtually any drug can be allergenic. The most common agents are: antibiotics, sulfonamides, p-aminosalicylic acid, oral antidiabetic agents (carbutamide, tolbutamide), local anesthetics (p-aminobenzoic acid ethyl ester, procaine), phenothiazines, barbiturates, hydantoin derivatives, carbamide, radiological contrast media containing iodine, aminophenazone, aniline derivatives (phenacetin), salicylic acid derivatives, quinine, quinidine, phenolphthalein, mercury compounds, antithyroid agents (thio-, methylthio-, propylthiouracil), arsenobenzene derivatives, and antihistaminics.

Food allergy

The most important *food allergens* are fish, crustaceans, pork, cow's milk, cheese, eggs, chocolate, honey, strawberries, nuts, corn, tomatoes and citrus fruits. Acute urticaria is often caused by these foods. Erythema multiforme, atopic dermatitis and acne vulgaris are occasionally related to food factors.

Contact allergy

Common *contact allergens* are chromates, nickel compounds, mercurial salts, arsenicals, aromatic amines (p-phenylene diamine, aniline), azo dyes, halogenated aromatic nitro- and amino-compounds, turpentine, divalent phenols bearing aliphatic substitutes, tetramethylthiuram disulfide, mercaptobenzothiazol, phenol, formaldehyde, resins, epoxy resins, methacrylates, thioglycollates, various cosmetics, pentadecylcatechol (poison ivy, poison oak, poison sumac) and exotic hardwoods.

Skin tests

Diagnosis of allergy is facilitated by a number of easily performed cutaneous tests. *Patch tests* are eminently useful in delayed reactions (contact dermatitis); they carry the slight risk of other local reactions and exacerbation of the existing contact dermatitis. The suspected allergen is applied in proper dilution to the back or upper arm for one to two days. A typical dermatitic reaction after 24 to 48 hours indicates a positive test. Patch tests should not be applied in acute stages of dermatitis. *Intradermal skin tests* for immediate reactions are difficult to interpret; systemic allergic reactions of other shock organs (e.g., bronchial asthma) cannot be avoided and may be fatal. Other methods, such as passive transfer of antibodies by the PRAUSNITZ-KÜSTNER technique, and the exposition test, should be performed only under the supervision of experienced physicians.

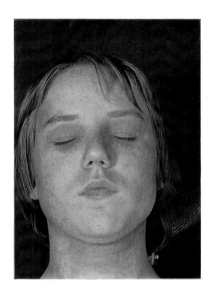

162

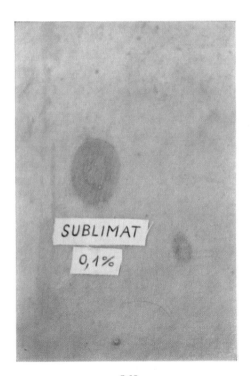

163

162 and **163**   **Contact dermatitis**
Induced by mercury ointment. Patch test positive after application
of 0.1 per cent mercuric chloride.

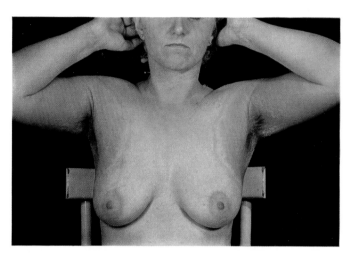

164 Allergic contact dermatitis
Induced by formalin impregnated garments.

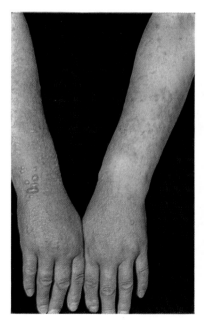

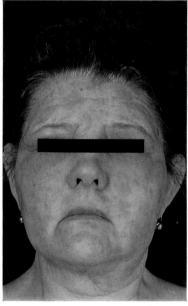

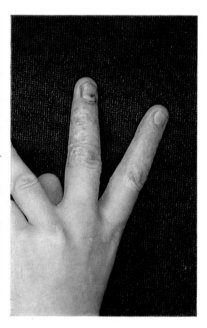

165 Allergic contact dermatitis
Bullous lesions on extensor surfaces of both arms due to penicillin ointment.

166 Allergic contact dermatitis
After topical application of penicillin ointment.

167 Allergic contact dermatitis
Occupational dermatitis in a physician, caused by procaine.

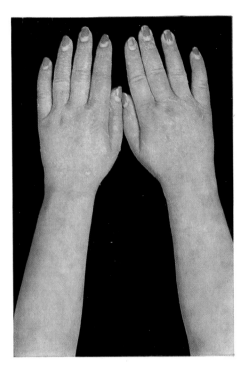

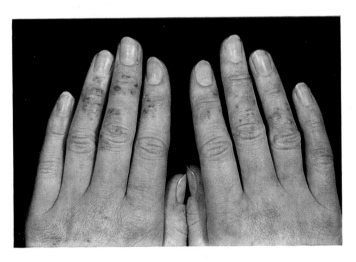

168   Allergic contact dermatitis
Erythema and scaling of both
forearms.

169   Allergic contact dermatitis
Occupational dermatitis in a beautician, caused by thio-
glycollate preparation.

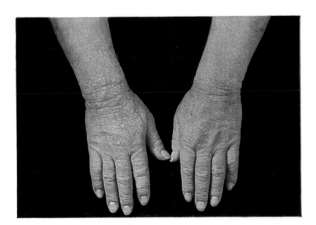

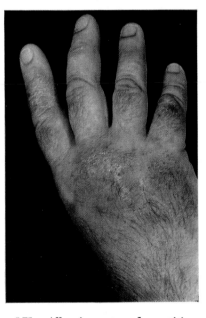

170   Allergic contact dermatitis
Occupational dermatitis due to cement
(chromates) in a bricklayer.
Chronic dry eczematous eruption of the hands.

171   Allergic contact dermatitis
Of the dorsum of the hand.

58

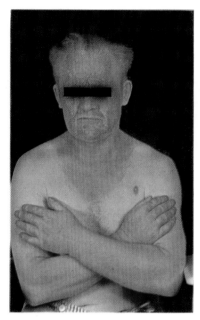

172 Allergic contact dermatitis
Due to Anaesthesin ointment.

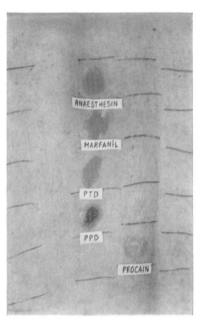

173 Positive patch test
To Anaesthesin and other substances with aromatic amino
groups in para-position (group
allergy).

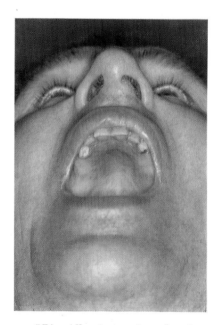

**174 Allergic reaction of oral
mucosa**
Induced by monomeric methacrylates (dentures).

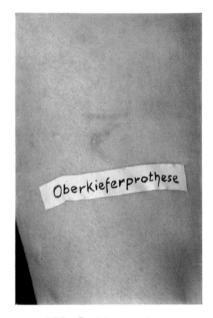

175 Positive patch test
Erythematous reaction due to
plastic component of dentures
(cf. fig. 172).

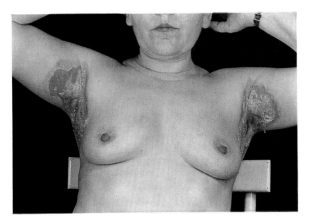

176 Allergic contact dermatitis
Due to dress shields (allergic reaction to rubber accelerators).

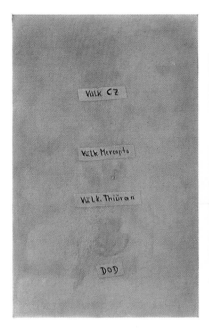

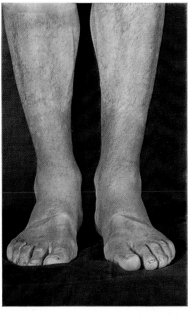

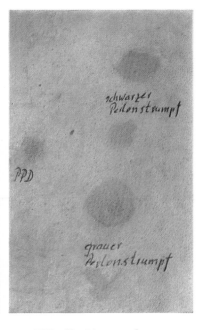

177 Positive patch test
Severe, partially bullous reaction to rubber accelerators.

178 Allergic contact dermatitis
Erythema and scaling of lower third of legs (contact with nylon-type stockings).

179 Positive patch test
To stockings of patient shown in figure 178.

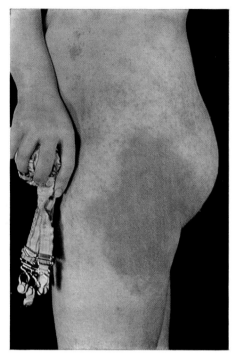

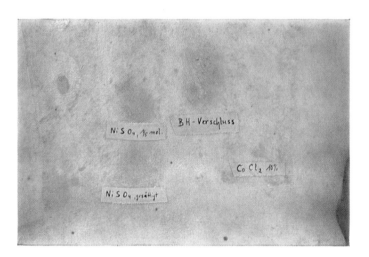

180   Allergic contact dermatitis
Due to nickel buckles.

181   Positive patch test
Group allergy to nickel sulfate (garter belt buckle)
and cobalt.

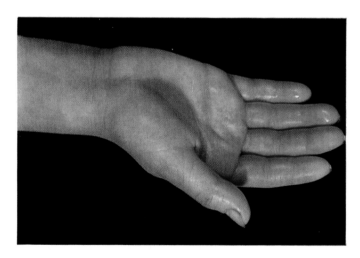

182   Typical "lacquer hand"
Occupational dermatosis of a beautician.

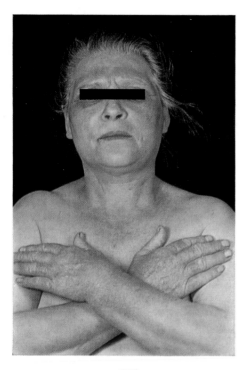

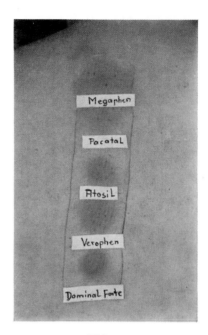

183 **184**

183 and 184   Contact dermatitis due to phenothiazine derivative
Positive patch test. Typical group allergy.

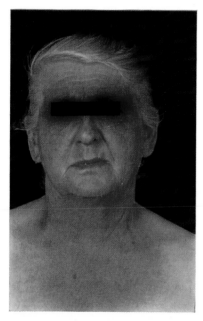

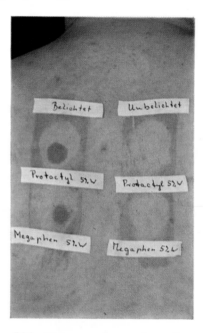

185   Allergic contact dermatitis
Marked erythema of face and neck due to a phenothiazine derivative.

186   Photo patch test in patient allergic to phenothiazines
While simple epicutaneous application of the agents caused no reaction (right side), marked localized erythema appeared after exposure to light (left side). (Photosensitizing effect of phenothiazines.)

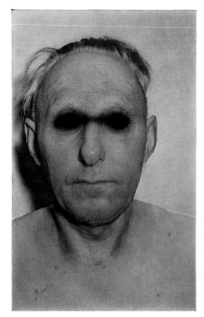

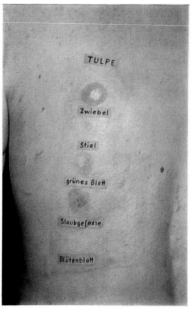

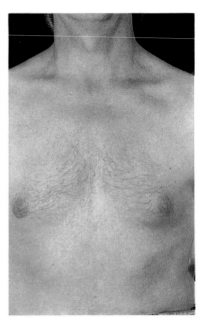

187 Allergic contact dermatitis
Due to plant allergens.

188 Patch test
Pertaining to figure 187. Frequently, only certain parts of the plant contain the allergen. Stamen, leaf, and bulb of the tulip produce a positive response, whereas the reaction to petal and stem is negative.

189 Scarlatiniform drug eruption
Due to systemic administration of penicillin.

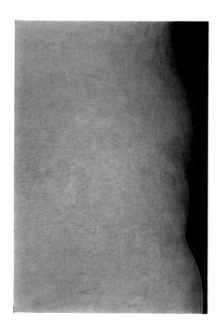

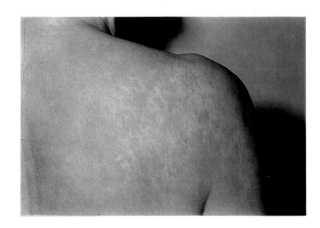

190 Morbilliform drug eruption
Due to parenteral administration of streptomycin.

191 Confluent maculopapular drug eruption
Due to sulfanylbutyl carbamide.

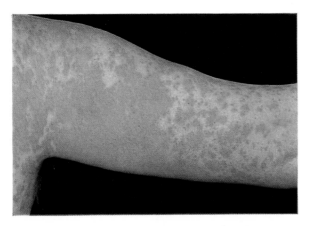

192   Confluent macular drug eruption
Due to a hydantoin derivative.

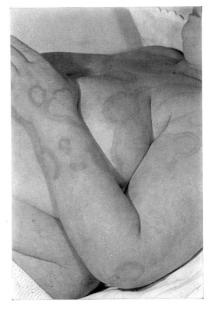

193   Urticaria
Due to parenteral administration
of penicillin.

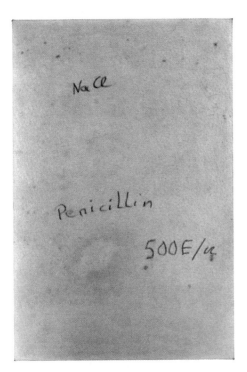

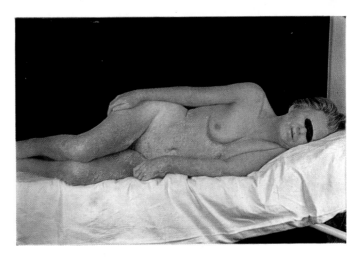

194   Positive intracutaneous test
Wheal with peripheral erythematous
flare and pseudopods following penicillin injection.

195   Severe exfoliative drug eruption (erythroderma)
Due to a pyrazolone derivative.

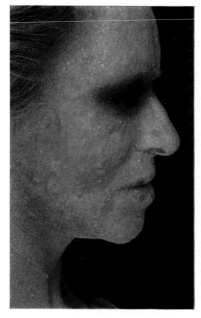

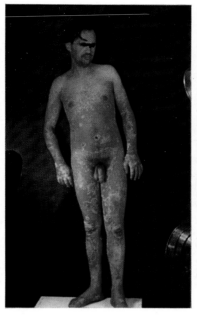

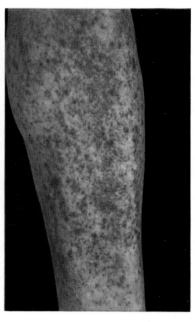

196 Exfoliative drug eruption
(Close-up view of figure 195)
Severe erythema, infiltration, and
scaling of facial skin.

**197 Severe erythrodermic drug
eruption**
Massive reaction following systemic administration of an anti-
psoriatic arsenic preparation in a
psoriatic patient.

198 Purpuric drug eruption
Following ingestion of a quinine-
containing anti-influenza drug.

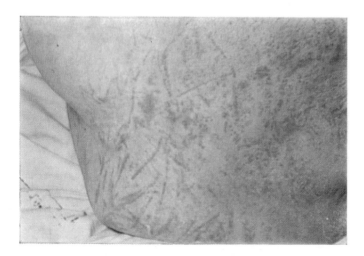

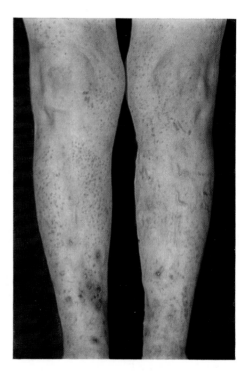

199 Thrombocytopenic purpura
Drug eruption due to thalidomide. The back shows numerous
linear petechiae caused by wrinkles in the bedsheet.

**200 Allergic vasculitis (Ruiter)
(drug eruption)**
Erythematous, purpuric, and necrotic
lesions of the lower leg.

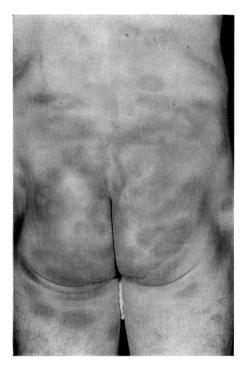

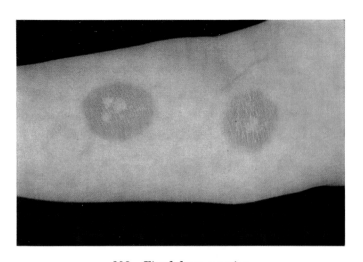

202 Fixed drug eruption
Due to analgesic containing pyrazolone. Round, erythematous, and hyperpigmented patches, recurrent in identical location.

201 Fixed drug eruption
Due to barbiturates.

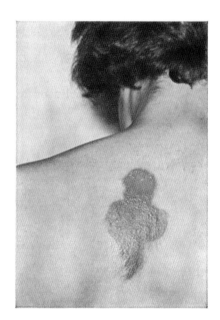

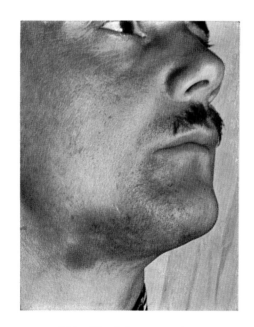

203 Fixed drug eruption
Persistent, sharply marginated, violaceous patch on back caused by weight control pills.

204 Fixed drug eruption
Recurrent hyperpigmented and erythematous eruption of chin area due to barbiturates.

Infectious Diseases of the Skin

Micrococcal Infections

Most purulent skin diseases are due to infections by streptococci or staphylococci. Principal portals of entry are the hair follicles in adults and the sweat ducts in infants and children. Lack of hygiene and increased perspiration due to high humidity produce epidermal changes which facilitate invasion by the micrococci. Lymphogenous and hematogenous infections are rare. Important factors determining the course and development of micrococcal infections of the skin are pathogenicity, virulence, and contagiosity of the microorganisms, and the predisposition or resistance of the host.

Pathogenic organisms can be identified by means of specific culture media, and their sensitivity to antibiotics can be determined by special techniques.

Classification of micrococcal skin diseases is a controversial problem. The most widely recognized systems are those of DARIER, who attempts to classify pyodermas according to the depth of the lesions, and of JADASSOHN, who takes into consideration etiology, relationship of the skin changes to the skin appendages, site of the lesions (epidermal, dermal, or hypodermal), and extent of the infection.

Follicular impetigo (BOCKHART)

This superficial micrococcal infection (usually due to coagulase-positive staphylococci, M. pyogenes var. aureus) is limited to the follicular ostia; it may be idiopathic, but more frequently it occurs as a complication of existing dermatoses, or after application of tar products, oils, and moist occlusive dressings.

The primary lesion is a pinhead-sized or larger, thin-walled, dome-shaped pustule filled with yellowish-green pus, often pierced by a hair and surrounded by a narrow, slightly infiltrated red halo; not infrequently, this primary lesion later develops into a furuncle. The disease can be differentiated from a deep folliculitis by the absence of edema, infiltration, and pain. Vacciniform pustulosis, a typical ostiofolliculitis, also belongs to this category.

Furuncle

A furuncle is a deep folliculitis and perifolliculitis of bacterial origin, with infiltration extending into the cutis and subcutis; this, in association with the concomitant edema, produces severe pain and tenderness. The furuncle may develop on the basis of a follicular impetigo, but more frequently it originates from a firm, painful infiltrate in the depth of the follicle. Systemic symptoms are rare. After perforation and discharge of the pus and central core (follicular and perifollicular necrosis), the furuncle eventually heals, leaving a scar.

Carbuncle

A carbuncle is formed by coalescing follicular and perifollicular necroses of several adjacent furuncles. The lesion is seen more frequently in older patients, predominantly in males. The local process is of considerable depth, the general health is sometimes impaired.

The appearance of furuncles or carbuncles immediately calls for measures to rule out diabetes mellitus.

Sycosis barbae (Folliculitis barbae)

This rare disorder is more common in bearded men. It presents an extremely polymorphous clinical picture. On a background of reddened, edematous skin, discrete papules or pustules, each pierced by a hair shaft and surrounded by an inflammatory halo, are seen next to erosions, perforated pustules discharging pus, and larger inflamed nodules from which hairs imbedded in a gelatinous mass may be plucked without pain.

The preferred area is the beard (barber's itch), but eyelashes, eyebrows, scalp, as well as axillary, pubic and body hair may also be involved. The causative organisms are usually staphylococci, sometimes streptococci. The disease does not tend to heal spontaneously; its therapy is time-consuming and taxes the patience of both physician and patient.

Acne keloid (Folliculitis keloidalis nuchae)
(Dermatitis papillaris capillitii (Kaposi))

Acne keloid is probably due to infection by M. pyogenes var. aureus and var. albus in association with individual and hormonal factors. The disease is predominant in males, particularly in Negroes. It usually affects the back of the neck with small follicular pustules, subcutaneous abscesses and hard keloidal papules. In its advanced stage it is characterized by transversally arranged irregular keloidal plaques and large cicatrized areas with isolated hair bundles (several hairs emerging from one follicular orifice).

Folliculitis decalvans (Brocq)

This rare chronic follicular eruption of the scalp may cause patchy cicatricial alopecia. The isolated or coalescent lesions are characterized by a slowly advancing irregular or gyrate border with follicular papules and pustules and an atrophic healed center. Coagulase-positive micrococci often can be demonstrated.

Perifolliculitis capitis abscedens et suffodiens (Hoffmann)
(Dissecting cellulitis of the scalp)

Indolent, moderately inflamed nodules undermine large areas of the scalp, form fluctuant abscesses and draining sinuses, and cause permanent alopecia of the affected areas. The lesions later coalesce to form irregular hypertrophic scars. The disease, which predominantly affects male Negroes, is often classified with acne conglobata and hidradenitis suppurativa as a variant of the follicular occlusion triad. The tendency to comedo formation, abscesses, sinuses, and healing with keloidal scars is characteristic of all three disorders, which often coexist in the same patient.

Although its relationship to acne vulgaris is unclarified, *acne conglobata* will be discussed in the chapter on acne.

Acne necrotica (Hebra)
(Acne varioliformis)

In contrast to acne vulgaris, this rare chronic, recurrent condition occurs in middle age; also in contrast, comedones or cysts are absent. On the forehead, the hairline, the temporal area, and the scalp (rarely on the face, chest, and back), discrete bright red papules and pustules appear, with a small disk-shaped necrotic area developing in the center. A round, depressed, superficial scar remains after the crust has fallen off. The lesions are not limited to the hair follicles. Bacteriologic examination regularly reveals staphylococci and streptococci.

Hidradenitis suppurativa
(Apocrine sweat gland abscesses)

Painful confluent abscesses of apocrine sweat glands of the axillary or anogenital region usually develop from small red nodular subcutaneous infiltrations or from a folliculitis. Coalescing nodules often form elongated masses parallel to the body folds, with purulent draining sinus tracts.

Pemphigus neonatorum (Impetigo neonatorum)

This rare, acute, often fatal bullous variety of impetigo occurs in infants in poor health in the postnatal period. In many cases, it can be traced to impetigo contagiosa of older siblings, or to paronychia of the person attending the infant.

Another rare variety of severe infantile pyoderma is *dermatitis exfoliativa neonatorum* (Ritter von Rittershain), which shows coalescent flaccid bullae, widespread exfoliation, and severe systemic symptoms.

Impetigo contagiosa

This common type of pyoderma is caused by various organisms. It is highly contagious only to infants and does not leave scars. Small yellow pustules with an intense erythematous base which dry up rapidly, leaving heavy, stuck-on, honey-colored crusts, are often caused by streptococci, whereas shallow, rapidly spreading bullae coalescing into circinate, fast-drying and scaling lesions with flat brownish crusts sometimes are due to staphylococci. However, mixed infections are more common.

Ecthyma

Ecthyma is a deep variety of impetigo. It is characterized by large erosive or ulcerative lesions covered with thick purulent crusts. These lesions are more common in areas with diminished blood supply or in debilitated patients.

Pityriasis alba faciei
(Furfuraceous impetigo)

Children and teenagers often show symmetrically arranged, discrete round scaling dry hypopigmented patches on both cheeks. The etiology of the disorder is unknown; it is more likely an early manifestation of seborrheic or atopic dermatitis than a superficial streptococcal infection as was originally assumed.

Erysipelas

This superficial streptococcal cellulitis starts with high temperatures and chills, and is characterized by tender, sharply circumscribed, shiny, hot, red, edematous plaques. The lesions spread with raised advancing borders and red lymphangitic streaks. Fever, malaise, and systemic symptoms are common but may be absent in older patients.

Vesicular, bullous, gangrenous, and phlegmonous variants of erysipelas also occur.

Chronic recurrent erysipelas (as well as recurrent thrombophlebitis) gradually leads to *elephantiasis nostras* which is characterized by a chronic lymphedema and pachyderma.

Bacterial paronychia

Purulent, recurrent, often chronic inflammation of the tissues around the nail frequently is due to prolonged maceration, or follows hangnails or vigorous manicuring of the nail folds. The disorder is more common in women. The nail folds are red, swollen, tense, and painful. In acute cases, a small amount of pus often can be expressed from the tender areas.

Chronic vegetating pyoderma
(Dermatitis vegetans)

Livid to reddish-brown edematous infiltrations, with exuberant granulation tissue, or papillary, verrucous, ulcerative, and draining moist vegetative plaques, ranging from coin to hand size, may develop as secondary infections of pre-existing eczematous regions, particularly in body folds, after injuries to the extremities, or on amputation stumps. Circulatory deficiency or chronic debilitating diseases are contributing factors.

Chancriform pyoderma (Hoffmann)

Round, oozing infiltrations with indolent swelling of regional lymph nodes may be located on the tongue, the lips, or the external genitals. The lesions heal spontaneously after 6 to 8 weeks. Darkfield examination and serologic tests to rule out syphilitic infection are indicated.

Bacillary Infections

Anthrax

Bacillus anthracis infections usually occur in cattle and sheep, but also in hogs, fowl, horses, and deer. Man is infected either by direct contact with these animals, or by handling their hides or contaminated soil. Occupations especially exposed to this infection are farmers, veterinarians, butchers, longshoremen, leather and wool handlers, laboratory personnel, and physicians.

After an incubation period of 2 to 8 days, a red maculopapular lesion appears at the portal of entry of the pathogenic organism (usually hands or fingers). Two days later, a flaccid, serous, later hemorrhagic bulla (*pustula maligna*) develops in the center of the lesion. The surrounding area becomes intensely infiltrated and shows a reddish-brown to livid coloring; the regional lymph nodes are enlarged. The center of the hemorrhagic bulla dries up to form a painless ulcer covered with a characteristic black adherent *eschar*. Occasionally, progressive edematous infiltrations lead to invasion of the blood stream by the organism. The resulting *septicemia* is associated with severe systemic manifestations, and has a grave prognosis. Patients afflicted with anthrax should be kept isolated.

Erysipeloid (ROSENBACH)

After an incubation period of 1 to 2 days, a typical violaceous to red, well defined, inflammatory edematous lesion appears at the site of inoculation with swine erysipelas (Erysipelothrix rhusiopathiae) following minor trauma to the hands or fingers. The lesions progress rapidly in arciform or gyrate configurations with a tendency to central clearing. The manifestations are considerably less acute than those of erysipelas. Systemic symptoms are usually absent; a generalized infection with endocarditis and joint pains is very rare. The disease is contracted through the handling of meat from infected animals, particularly fish, shellfish, venison or poultry, or through contact with decaying wood or contaminated soil.

Cutaneous Leishmaniasis (Oriental sore, Aleppo boil)

After an incubation period of a few days to several months, the protozoal parasite (Leishmania tropica), usually transmitted by mosquito bites (Phlebotomus sandflies), produces small, itching, purple papules which gradually develop into nodules or indurated disk-like lesions with brownish marginal zones. Sharply circumscribed, round punched-out ulcers with indurated borders are frequently seen. Infiltrated lesions may simulate a syphilitic chancre; crusted ulcers are suggestive of pyodermas. The disease is common in the Middle East and in tropical areas of Asia, Africa, and America. It is limited to the skin and occurs principally on exposed areas of children and young adults. Spontaneous remission often occurs after several months, leaving immunity. Diagnostic tests include demonstration of the parasite in smears obtained by curetting, and a delayed response to the leishmanin test.

Mucocutaneous leishmaniasis
(South American leishmaniasis)

This tropical disease caused by Leishmania brasiliensis is predominant in South America, particularly in wooded regions. The skin lesions resemble those of cutaneous leishmaniasis; in addition, there is a moderate tendency to involve the mucous menbranes of nose, mouth and pharynx. The diagnosis is established by skin scrapings and a delayed reaction to the Montenegro test.

Tuberculosis of the Skin

Cutaneous tuberculosis rarely is seen in the United States of America.

All skin changes produced by Mycobacterium tuberculosis (KOCH) are referred to as tuberculosis of the skin. Bacteriologic examination of the lesions usually reveals the human, less frequently the bovine type of the mycobacterium. Despite their common etiology, the clinical manifestations of cutaneous tuberculosis vary widely due to different allergic responses.

The course of the disease depends largely on the patient's biologic reactions. This specific allergy is easily determined by percutaneous and intracutaneous tests (VON PIRQUET, MORO, MENDEL-MANTOUX). The following responses are possible:

Anergic response

The organism fails to form antibodies either because it has not yet had contact with mycobacteria, or because it has exhausted its resources (cachexia). Invasion and propagation of the bacteria are not checked by the patient's defense mechanisms. Tuberculin reaction is negative.

Normergic response

Antibody formation of intermediate intensity signifies an equilibrium of host and pathogenic organism. Tuberculin reaction is positive ($1:10^4$).

Hyperergic response

The pathogen produces violent acute inflammatory reactions to the point of ulceration and necrosis. Tuberculin reaction is strongly positive (up to $1:10^7$).

Other factors determining the clinical course of skin tuberculosis are the pathways used by the mycobacterium (disseminated through blood or lymph channels, by contiguity or exogenous infection) and the zone of the skin where the microorganism eventually settles.

Primary inoculation tuberculosis

The tuberculous primary complex (tuberculous chancre) of the skin, consisting of a nodule slowly evolving into an indurated ulcer, occurs almost exclusively in infants and young children. Areas of predilection are the face and extremities. Prominent regional lymphadenopathy is a characteristic finding. The incubation period is 2 to 4 weeks. BCG vaccination also may produce the picture of a cutaneous tuberculous primary complex.

Tuberculosis cutis orificialis
(Tuberculosis ulcerosa cutis et mucosae)

In a completely anergic state (negative tuberculin test), highly contagious, rapidly ulcerating, indolent skin lesions may occur in the preterminal stage of visceral tuberculosis, involving areas contiguous to mucocutaneous junctions. These lesions are produced by massive auto-inoculation of mycobacteria excreted with body fluids.

Lupus vulgaris (Tuberculosis cutis luposa)

This is the most common form of cutaneous tuberculosis, manifesting a normergic state of allergy. It can be produced only by superinfection, usually endogenously, i.e., by hematogenous dissemination. In the course of months or years, an isolated, soft, red or yellowish-brown nodule slowly develops into the characteristic chronic annular scaling plaque. The diagnostically significant nodule, occuring primarily on the face, is comprised histologically of a collection of typical tubercles. On diascopic examination, the area is blanched, revealing pinhead-sized round nodules of apple-jelly color. With a fine probe, the necrotic infiltrate is easily penetrated; the resulting bleeding ceases readily.

Different clinical types of lupus vulgaris are described in the legends to the illustrations.

Scrofuloderma (Tuberculosis cutis colliquativa)

A form of cutaneous tuberculosis based on a normergic response in children, scrofuloderma usually derives from a tuberculous infection of the lymph nodes or bones underlying the affected skin area. Less frequently, primary subcutaneous lesions are produced by hematogenous dissemination. Characteristic clinical features are slowly enlarging lymph nodes (usually of the neck) which gradually become adherent to the skin, necrotize, and discharge thin yellowish-green pus through fistulous openings, leaving bizarre corded hypertrophic scars.

Tuberculosis verrucosa cutis

This condition, which is also called "prosector's wart," usually occurs in the hands and has its highest incidence in persons handling tuberculous material (pathologists, veterinarians, butchers, etc.). The lesions are produced by exogenous infection in a normergic state of allergy. They start as red papules which become crusted and may develop into large vegetative, verrucous plaques with slight purulent discharge.

Tuberculids

In a markedly hyperergic state of allergy, hematogenous dissemination may produce symmetrically arranged lesions referred to as tuberculids (DARIER). Demonstration of mycobacteria in the skin has been reported. Local circulatory deficiencies may play a significant pathogenetic rôle in *erythema induratum Bazin* and *papulonecrotic tuberculids*. Other tuberculids are *lichen scrofulosorum (tuberculosis cutis lichenoides)* and *tuberculosis miliaris disseminata faciei*. In rare cases, tuberculids may simulate granuloma annulare, erythema nodosum, or lichen nitidus.

Lichen scrofulosorum (HEBRA)
(Tuberculosis cutis lichenoides)

Small, skin-colored or pink to reddish-brown, flat-topped, firm follicular papules appear at first in scattered isolated lesions, later as patches or lichenoid papules, on the trunk of children with systemic tuberculosis. The lichenoid lesions often bear fine scales or horny plugs. Spontaneous remissions and recurrences have been reported.

Papulonecrotic tuberculid
(Tuberculosis papulonecrotica)

Indolent purplish papules, pustules, necroses, and varioliform scars on the extensor aspects of the distal extremities or the face are typical of this disorder, which often takes a chronic, recurrent course. The disease occurs in adults with an active form of tuberculosis elsewhere, indicating a hyperergic response.

Erythema induratum (BAZIN)
(Tuberculosis indurativa cutanea et subcutanea)

This type of hyperergic tuberculosis of the skin occurs most commonly in younger women with peripheral circulatory disorders. Solitary or grouped indolent nodular infiltrates are localized on the borderline between cutis and subcutis, especially of the calves of the legs. The overlying skin turns bluish-red, the lesions ulcerate and eventually heal with scar formation. Usually, all stages of the chronic recurrent disease are seen simultaneously in one patient.

Some authors consider the DARIER-ROUSSY type of sarcoidosis a variety of tuberculosis indurativa; in this disorder, the skin over the deep subcutaneous infiltrates is not discolored, but it is adherent to the underlying tissue. The symmetrically arranged lesions may involve any part of the integument. Ulceration does not occur. After healing of the lesions, the skin may show crateriform depressions.

Lupus miliaris disseminatus faciei
(TILBURY-FOX)

(Tuberculosis miliaris disseminata faciei)

Small, soft, noncoalescing dome-shaped papules of pale red to yellowish-brown or brownish-red coloring occur bilaterally, mainly in the face of adult patients. Diascopy shows "apple jelly" infiltrates. The papular lesions may heal with scar formation. Clinically, this rare disorder is more closely related to papulonecrotic tuberculid than to lupus vulgaris, and may therefore be classified as a tuberculid. The immunobiological state associated with this disease also suggests its relationship to the tuberculid group.

Leprosy (HANSEN)

This mildly contagious, chronic infectious disease, which has been known for several millenia, is caused by Mycobacterium leprae (HANSEN). Millions are still suffering from this disease, though it is rare in the United States. Two clinical types are known. The more malignant, contagious *lepromatous leprosy* (nodular leprosy), is characterized by nodular infiltrates (lepromas), which often start as erythematous macules with diffuse borders. These macules are localized mostly on the ear lobes, nose, supraorbital region (leonine facies), elbows, and buttocks. Scrapings of these lesions show mycobacteria in great numbers. The nasal mucous membranes become involved at an early stage of the disease; the lepromas ulcerate, causing epistaxis, perforation of the septum, and further dissemination of the organisms with the nasal secretions. Internal organs, lymph nodes, eyes, and bones also may become involved. Necrotic sequestration and mutilation may occur, especially on the hands and feet. The lepromin (Mitsuda) reaction is negative (anergic response). Erythema nodosum-like reactions are common.

The second, more frequent, and relatively benign type, *tuberculoid leprosy* (maculo-anesthetic leprosy), is noninfectious and may heal spontaneously if living conditions are adequate. Large erythemato-squamous, slightly raised, often circinate anhidrotic plaques are arranged in an asymmetrical pattern on the face, extremities, and buttocks. The sharply outlined anesthetic macular lesions are often hypopigmented and show central clearing. Involvement of the mucous membranes is rare. Progressive neurological involvement with neuritis and fusiform thickening of ulnar and peroneal nerves is typical. The disease does not spread to internal organs. The lepromin test is positive; bacilli cannot always be demonstrated.

Atypical forms of an intermediate nature are referred to as *indeterminate types of leprosy*. The Mitsuda reaction may be negative or positive. Mycobacteria are sparse or absent. The *borderline* or *dimorphic type* is not stable and may change into other types.

Fungal diseases of the skin
(Dermatomycoses) (VIRCHOW)

Infectious diseases of the skin, hair, and nails, when produced essentially by ringworm fungi and yeasts, are referred to as dermatomycoses. The causative organisms are easily demonstrable microscopically. Examination of scrapings treated with 10 per cent potassium hydroxide yields positive results in a high percentage of cases. Hyphae and spores can be visualized; however, identification of the type of fungus, or even differentiation between dermatophytes and yeasts, is not possible by this method. This must be done with the aid of special culture media.

Tineas (Dermatophytoses)

Fungi penetrating into the upper epidermal layers produce a small, red, itching and scaling spot which grows centrifugally. The marginal zone of the lesion is occupied by numerous small vesicles which soon become pustular. While the central portion of the eruption tends to heal spontaneously, the raised marginal zone spreads in a ring-like pattern. An obsolete term for superficial tineas is trichophytia superficialis, which was used to differentiate it from deeper dermatophytic infections (tinea profunda, trichophytia profunda).

Tineas involving deeper layers of the skin usually develop from longstanding superficial tineas. Ostiofollicular pustules, folliculitis, perifolliculitis, and necrotic degeneration may occur. The lesions coalesce into verruciform or dome-shaped, soft succulent tumors. Upon application of pressure, pus drains from numerous openings as from a sponge. In the past, this type was often seen in the beard area (sycosis barbae).

Deep follicular fungus infections of the lower legs are often seen in women after they have shaved their legs. They are characterized by livid, itching, nodular granulomas which may extend into the subcutaneous tissue. Hyphae and spores are usually demonstrable when affected hairs are treated with potassium hydroxide.

Some special clinical types of tineas, which are due to regional differences, will be discussed in greater detail.

Tinea unguium (Onychomycosis)

This infection usually involves a single nail, rarely all of the fingernails or toenails. The dermatophytes grow in the nail plate, which becomes opaque, brittle, cracked, and partially separated from the nail bed, and shows a dirty yellowish-gray discoloration. The nail infection is usually associated with a fungus infection of the surrounding skin (frequently caused by Trichophyton rubrum).

Tinea cruris (Tinea marginatum Hebra)

This chronic pruritic fungus infection, which spreads peripherally in polycyclic configurations with a slightly elevated border and scaling center, occurs predominantly in the genitocrural area. The fungi most frequently isolated from these lesions are Trichophyton rubrum, Trichophyton mentagrophytes, and Epidermophyton floccosum.

Tinea pedis et manua

This infection of the hands and feet is often caused by trichophyton species. Clinically, a dyshidrotic, a squamous-hyperkeratotic and an intertriginous type can be distinguished.

Dermatophytids

Sudden macular, lichenoid, or vesicular eruptions may be associated with systemic symptoms (fever, chills, headaches) as the result of a hyperergic state of allergy. The trichophytin test is strongly positive in dilutions up to 1:300. Another important criterion for the diagnosis of a dermatophytid is the presence of an acute inflammatory infection elsewhere.

Dyshidrosis (Tilbury-Fox) and *Cheiropompholyx* (Hutchinson) are vesicular to bullous skin changes occuring on the hands in recurrent episodes; in many cases, they are considered dermatophytids. In most of the patients affected with this disorder, an acute interdigital tinea pedum will be found. Therapeutic efforts must be concentrated on the latter. *Dyshidrosis lamellosa sicca* is another form of dyshidrosis with subliminal vesiculation.

Tinea favosa (Schönlein)
(Favus)

Favus is caused by Trichophyton Schönleini (Achorion Schönleini). The characteristic yellow scutula (cup-shaped follicular crusts) have a fairly typical mousy odor. They produce flat, depressed scars in the affected scalp areas. Favus is extremely rare in the continental United States.

Tinea capitis

Tinea capitis used to occur epidemically in children. The scalp shows round or oval, sharply defined lesions covered with pityriasiform scales. In the affected area, the hairs are broken off at a length of about 1 mm.

In rare cases, the skin is reddened or moderately infiltrated. In addition to the scalp, skin areas covered with vellus hair and nails may be affected. Under Wood's light, the tinea lesions or epilated hairs infested with the fungus show a typical bright yellowish-green fluorescence. The infection may be caused by Microsporum audouini, M. canis (often contracted from animals), or M. gypseum. *Kerion celsi* occurs as an allergic reaction in severe cases of tinea capitis in form of sharply defined partially alopecic soft succulent granulomatous areas with numerous purulent draining openings.

Tinea versicolor (Pityriasis versicolor)

This frequently encountered superficial fungus infection caused by Malassezia furfur is even more common in hot, humid climates. Sharply defined confluent, round or irregular, yellowish to brownish or depigmented, slightly scaling patches usually involve the upper trunk, neck, and upper arms. The scaling becomes more evident after gentle scraping.

Erythrasma

Small, red, sharply defined lesions, coalescing into brownish or reddish-brown patches with very faint scaling, are seen on the inner aspect of the thighs adjacent to the scrotum or labia, in the axillary and submammary areas and between the fourth and fifth toes. The involved areas show coral red fluorescence under Wood's light. The causative organism was originally named Nocardia minutissima; it can be visualized under oil immersion. Recent investigations indicate that it is a bacterium and not a fungus.

Candidiasis (Moniliasis)

Yeast infections have gained increasing clinical importance in recent years. Diseases caused by yeasts and yeast-like fungi are common in intertriginous areas; they also can involve mucous membranes and internal organs. Interdigital monilial infections of the toes and onychomycosis of the toes and fingers cannot be distinguished clinically from similar dermatoses caused by dermatophytes. Differentiation of the microorganisms is possible only by the use of culture media.

Typical yeast infections of the skin are *interdigital moniliasis* (erosio interdigitalis blastomycetica), *monilial intertrigo, monilial paronychia, thrush* (moniliasis of the mouth), and *monilial vaginitis. Monilial granulomas* rarely occur on skin and mucous membranes. Id reactions (candidids) are not uncommon.

Chromoblastomycosis

This disease is seen mainly in tropical and subtropical climates. Ulcerated, verrucous or papillomatous growths form on a papular base, especially on the lower extremities. The causative organisms (Phialophora verrucosa, Hormodendrum pedrosoi, Hormodendrum compactum, and other fungi) invade the tissue through small abrasions. They are easily demonstrable in smears and histologic preparations.

Mycetoma
(Madura foot) (Carter and Colebrook)

Mycetoma or Madura mycosis is characterized by tumorous, draining, subcutaneous infiltrations of the feet induced by actinomycetes, ascomycetes and fungi imperfecti. The disease occurs chiefly in tropical and subtropical regions, but may be encountered elsewhere.

Actinomycosis

Actinomyces israeli, the microorganism causing actinomycosis, is a bacterial organism rather than a fungus. The chronic infiltrating inflammatory process is most common in the cervico-facial area, starting on the oral mucosa or the tonsils. Other forms involve the thoracic or abdominal area. Characteristic clinical features are mildly tender woody induration, abscess formation, ulceration, sinus tracts, and purulent discharge. The diagnosis is confirmed by the presence of tiny whitish or yellowish "sulfur granules" (masses of fungi) which often can be visualized macroscopically.

Viral diseases of the skin

Viruses cannot be cultured in synthetic media; they multiply only in living cells. Dermatologic research has yielded considerable insight into the various types of viruses and their relationship to the host cells. Virus diseases occur in men, in animals, and in plants; the size of the individual virus ranges from 10 to 300 mμ. They cannot be visualized with the light microscope; their morphological characteristics have been investigated by means of electron microscopy. Chemically, they consist of nucleic acid and protein. The elementary bodies of the infected cells are the carriers of infectiosity. Viruses producing pathologic skin changes primarily in men are those causing molluscum contagiosum, verrucae, condyloma acuminatum, herpes simplex, zoster, varicellae, variola vera, vaccinia, milker's nodules, foot and mouth disease, cat scratch disease, various exanthematous infectious diseases, and lymphogranuloma venereum (NICOLAS-FAVRE).

Viruses are cultivated most successfully when inoculated into chicken eggs.

Molluscum contagiosum (BATEMAN)

After an incubation period of 2 weeks to several months, discrete pinhead-sized, slowly growing, umbilicated, globular papules develop predominantly on the face (cheeks, eyelids and forehead), neck, and external genitals and surrounding areas of children. They may become inflamed and grow to pea-size or larger. Dense crops may form reddish-brown, verrucous lesions, with the central depression still visible. When compressed laterally, the eruptions discharge a cheesy white granular core through their central depressions. Mollusca involving the eyelids occasionally reach considerable size. They may cause stubborn conjunctivitis.

Warts

Verruca vulgaris, verruca plana juvenilis, verruca plantaris, and condyloma acuminatum are contagious, virus-induced tumors. The contagiosity of warts was recognized as early as 1896 (JADASSOHN). Incubation periods range from 4 weeks to 20 months. The same type of virus has been isolated from the morphologically widely differing lesions mentioned above. The clinical appearance of the verrucous tumors seems to be determined by the site on which they grow.

Verrucae planae juveniles (flat warts)

Flat, polygonal, skin-colored or slightly yellowish to reddish-brown papules develop on the dorsal aspects of fingers and hands, on the distal portions of the forearms, and in the face. Flat warts are seen predominantly in children and young adults. They appear suddenly and in great numbers, are often persistent, but may disappear just as suddenly and spontaneously. This is probably the reason they sometimes respond well to hypnosis.

Verrucae vulgares

These differ from flat warts by their size, their rough horny surface, and their predilection for the hands. *Periungual* and *plantar warts* are especially troublesome. On the eyelids, in the beard area, and on the lips, the verrucae develop as threadlike tumors and are therefore referred to as *filiform warts*.

Condylomata acuminata (Venereal warts)

Multiple soft, moist, reddish or skin-colored, pedunculated, small papillary tumors, often coalescing into large tumors with cauliflower-like surface, may involve the entire genital or anal region. They grow primarily on moist, macerated skin (vaginal discharge, phimosis, balanitis) and are sometimes venereal in origin.

Epidermodysplasia verruciformis (LEWANDOWSKY-LUTZ)

This disorder shows numerous verrucous lesions of different morphology, particularly on the dorsa of the hands and feet, on the face and on the neck. Positive inoculation experiments suggest that it is a generalized verrucosis, not a different disease entity. Some authors believe it to be an autosomal recessive precancerous genodermatosis.

Herpes simplex

This eruption, which is preceded by mild itching or burning, consists of grouped vesicles of uniform size on an erythematous base, involving the skin and mucous membranes. According to its localization, herpes is denoted as *herpes facialis, labialis, progenitalis, or digitalis (herpetic "whitlow")*. When the vesicles break, small superficial ulcers form on the skin and mucous membranes. Recurrent episodes are typical of herpes simplex. Regular recurrences at the same site are called herpes recidivans in loco. The causative organism, a virus, can be inoculated into the rabbit cornea, producing a punctate keratitis. A smear from the base of the vesicle (TZANCK test) shows multinucleated giant cells. Outbreak of the disease appears to be dependent on certain precipitating factors, such as menstruation, traumatization, sunlight exposure, gastrointestinal upsets, and psychological influences. Herpes simplex may also occur, in the form of typical *fever blisters* or *cold sores*, associated with febrile disorders. These different herpetic infections develop in patients with antibodies who were exposed to the virus before. Typical primary forms of herpes in patients without antibodies are *acute primary herpetic gingivostomatitis*, clinically presenting as *aphthous stomatitis, acute herpetic vulvovaginitis* and *acute herpetic kerato-conjunctivitis*. They are usually seen in children. Transmission of the infection may be exogenous or hematogenous. The incubation period is 2 to 5 days.

Eczema herpeticum

This disease is also known as KAPOSI's varicelliform eruption. It is a grave complication of eczematous eruptions, particularly of atopic dermatitis. It is characterized by numerous vesicles and pustules of uniform size superimposed on the pre-existing dermatosis, involvement of the oral mucosa, and dendritic keratitis. The disease is fatal in 10 per cent of adult patients and in 20 per cent of infants.

Zoster (SHINGLES)

Zoster is a unilateral, often band-like vesicular eruption on an erythemato-edematous base, situated along the distribution of nerves from one or several posterior ganglia. The disease produces immunity.

The grouped vesicular lesions later become purulent and umbilicated. *Hemorrhagic zoster* is characterized by hemorrhagic vesicles; *necrotic* or *gangrenous zoster* by necrotic degeneration of the base of the vesicles. Severe, burning neuritic pain may precede, accompany, or follow the outbreak of shingles, especially in older patients. Sensory impairment and transient muscle paresis may occur. The cerebrospinal fluid often shows increase in protein content and cell count. A smear from the base of the lesions shows multinucleated giant cells. The causative organism is similar to or identical with the varicella virus. The disease may occur as a complication of leukemia, HODGKIN's disease, internal cancer, administration of arsenicals, or carbon monoxide poisoning.

Varicella (Chickenpox)

In this febrile disease, pink macules develop into papules and then into pinhead- to lentil-sized, clear, tense, sometimes umbilicated vesicles on an erythematous base. They become purulent and eventually dry out with crust formation. The first lesions appear on face and back; later the eruption becomes generalized. New crops of vesicles may appear repeatedly, associated with elevated temperatures. Simultaneous existence of various developmental stages of varicella (macules, papules, vesicles, pustules, crusts) and involvement of the oral mucosa (especially the hard palate) are characteristic features. Varicella usually affects children, but adults also may contract the disease, which produces immunity. The TZANCK test shows multinucleated giant cells.

Variola vera (Smallpox)

The initial stage of this infection, following an incubation period of 8 to 12 days, is characterized by a 3-day period of fever, severe headache, backache, and vomiting. In most cases, a transient macular rash appears on the face and arms. The fever subsides after 3 days. Starting on the fifth day approximately, the exanthem is transformed into firm papules, then into vesicles, and finally into the typical umbilicated pustules on an erythematous base (suppurative stage); simultaneously, the temperature rises again. This stage is completed on or about the eighth day. The exanthem is generalized, with special emphasis on the face, arms, and palms. Particularly dense aggregates are seen in the vicinity of scar tissue or pressure areas. The oral mucosa shows ulcerating vesicles. On the twelfth day, the pustules begin to dry. The crusts are shed after 1 to $1\frac{1}{2}$ weeks, and scars remain. In the presence of hemorrhagic pustules or coalescing lesions (variola confluens), the prognosis is grave. Characteristically, all lesions of variola vera are in the same stage of development simultaneously.

Vaccinia

Prophylaxis against smallpox is based on vaccination with vaccinia lymph. JENNER originally used cowpox lymph (1796). Both viruses are closely related but not identical.

Dermatologically important complications of smallpox vaccination are *accidental vaccination* (autoinoculation of other areas of the body), *inoculation vaccinia* (transmission to noninoculated persons), and *eczema vaccinatum*.

Eczema vaccinatum

This disease is caused by inoculation of the vaccinia virus into skin altered by pre-existing eczematous conditions, particularly atopic dermatitis. This complication, as well as eczema herpeticum, was included in the older term "Kaposi's varicelliform eruption." After an incubation period of 5 to 12 days, the disease runs a predictable febrile course, regardless of the site of infection. From the face, where the changes are most marked, multiple umbilicated pustules spread centrifugally over the entire integument, sometimes healing with cicatrization.

Cowpox and Milker's nodules

The cowpox virus may be transmitted to man directly from infected teats and udders. The infection results in the formation of localized firm bluish-red nodules and pustules.

The paravaccinia virus is transferred from the cow's udder to the milker's hands where it produces nontender, firm, dome-shaped, yellowish-gray to bluish-red, pea-sized nodules which are called milker's nodules.

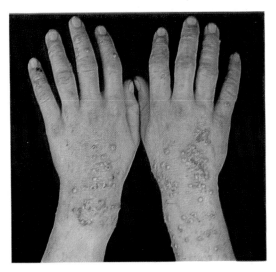

205 Follicular impetigo (Bockhart)

Superficial ostiofolliculitis confined to the hair
follicles. Each of the centrally depressed lesions
is pierced by a hair.

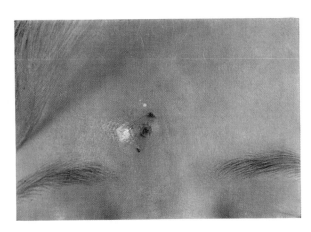

206 Furuncle shortly before perforation

Tender, erythematous, edematous infiltration
with central necrotic core.

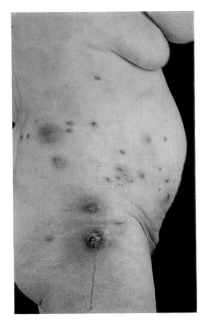

207 Furunculosis

Multiple, painful, draining
furuncles in a diabetic patient.

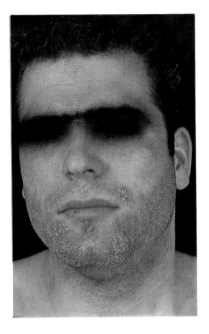

208 Sycosis (folliculitis) barbae

Beard area studded with small
follicular erythematous pustules.

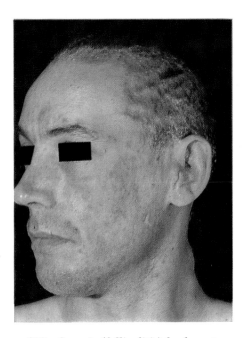

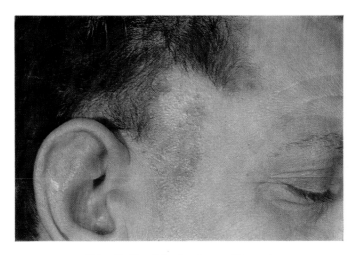

210   Folliculitis decalvans (BROCQ)

Follicular lesions healing with atrophy and partial alopecia.
A relationship to pseudopelade (BROCQ) is possible.

209   Sycosis (folliculitis) barbae et capillitii

Erythematous pustules of beard area
and scalp.

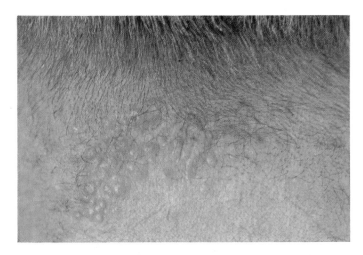

211   Acne keloid (folliculitis keloidalis nuchae)

Numerous erythematous papules (each pierced by a small
hair) and hard keloidal lesions.

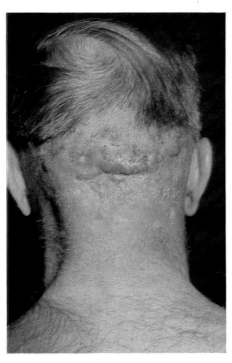

212   Acne keloid (folliculitis keloidalis nuchae)

Terminal stage, with irregularly shaped
transverse firm keloidal tumors of the
skin.

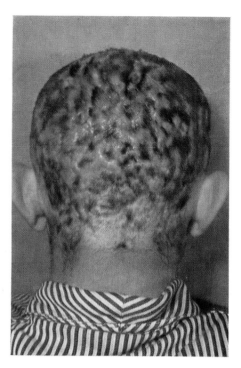

**213   Folliculitis et perifolliculitis abscedens et suffodiens
(dissecting cellulitis of the scalp)**
Fluctuant abscesses and draining sinuses healing with irregular hypertrophic scars.

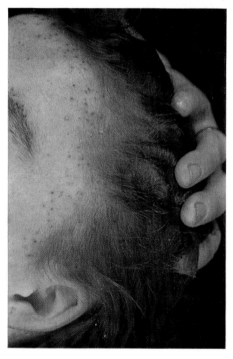

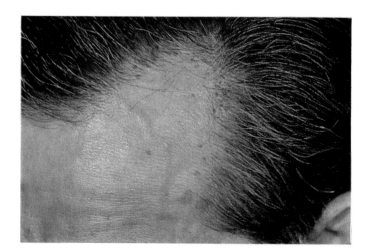

214   **215**

214 and 215   Acne necroticans (acne varioliformis)
Recurrent, discrete. red papules and pustules healing with small depressed scars.

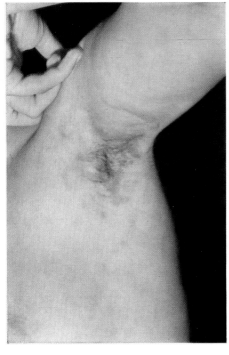

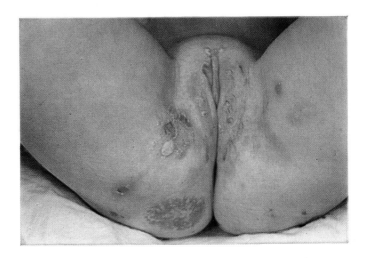

216   Hidradenitis suppurativa

Abscesses of apocrine sweat glands. Painful confluent lesions of axilla with purulent draining sinus tracts.

217   Bullous impetigo

In a 5-year-old girl. Large purulent bullae and pustules.

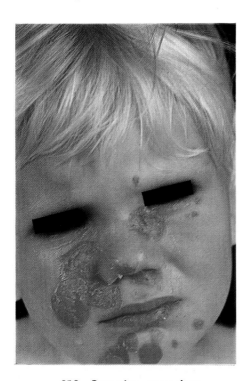

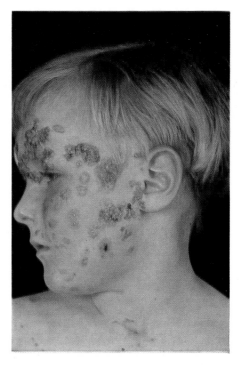

218   Impetigo contagiosa

Rapidly spreading circinate erythematous lesions with thick, shiny crusts and isolated vesicles; caused by staphylococci.

219   Impetigo contagiosa

New lesions covered with heavy, stuck-on, grayish-brown and honey-colored crusts; caused by streptococci. Older healing lesions.

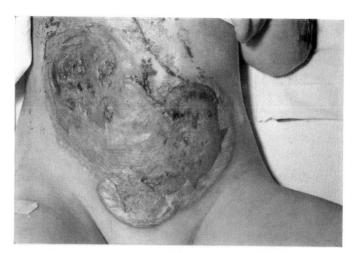

220   Progressive postoperative gangrene (CULLEN)
Probably of microbial origin, following appendectomy.

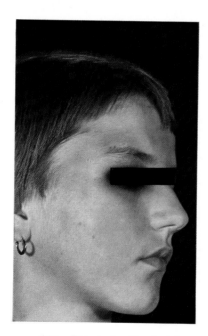

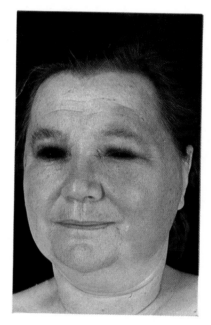

**221   Pityriasis alba faciei
(Furfuraceous impetigo)**
Dry hypopigmented patches with
fine furfuraceous scaling on
cheeks.

222   Erysipelas
Sharply circumscribed, tender,
hot, red, edematous area with
advancing raised border.

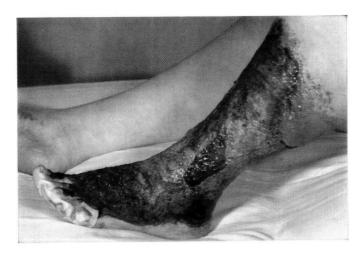

223   Hemorrhagic and gangrenous erysipelas of the lower leg
With sharply marginated raised border.

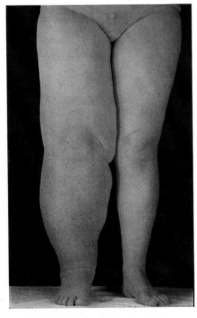

224   Elephantiasis nostras
Following chronic recurrent
erysipelas of the right leg.

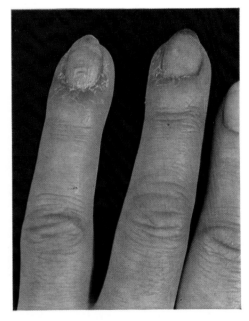

225   Chronic bacterial paronychia
Erythema, infiltration, scaling, and tenderness of nail fold with slight purulent
discharge and secondary dystrophic
changes of nail plate.

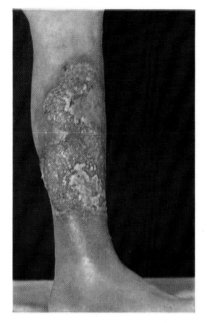

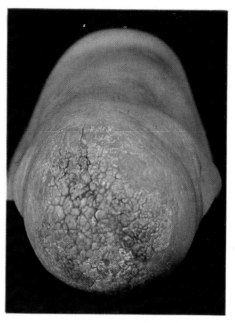

**226 Chronic vegetating pyoderma
(Dermatitis vegetans)**
Livid to reddish-brown edematous
infiltration with exuberant
vegetating granulation tissue.

227   Chronic vegetating pyoderma
On amputation stump.

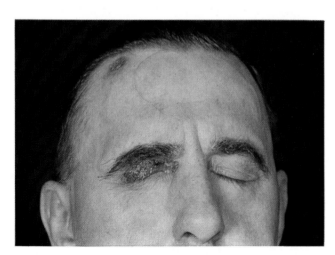

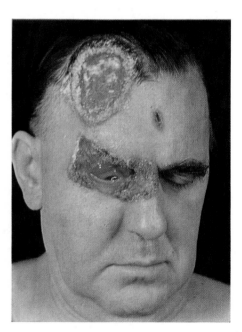

228   **229**

228 and 229   Chronic vegetating pyoderma
Early and advanced stages of a therapy-resistant case of several years' duration.

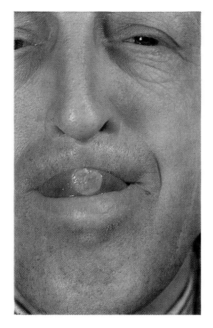

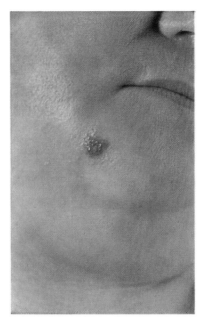

230   Chancriform pyoderma
(HOFFMANN)

Round, edematous, whitish infiltration of tongue suggestive of
primary syphilis; darkfield and
serologic test for syphilis (S.T.S.)
negative.

231   Anthrax (malignant pustule)

Flaccid, serosanguineous bulla.

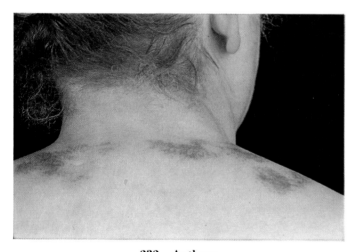

232   Anthrax

Edematous, phlegmonous, hemorrhagic lesions
of the upper back in the same patient.

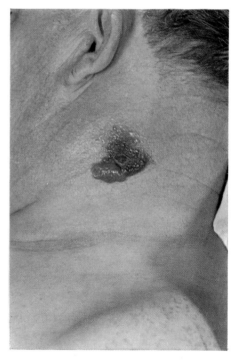

233   Anthrax (malignant pustule)

Formation of a black eschar over the
drying hemorrhagic bulla with infiltration of the surrounding tissue.

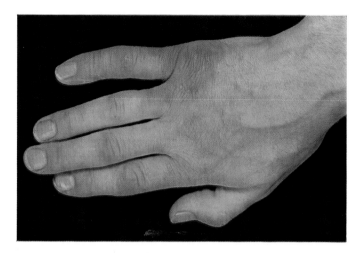

234 Erysipeloid (ROSENBACH)

Well defined, violaceous-red, edematous infiltration with arciform advancing border.

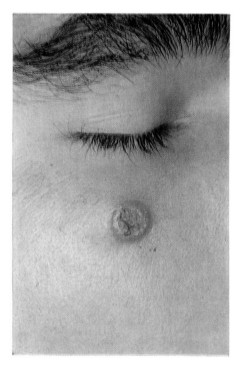

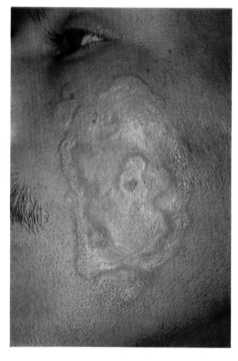

235   Cutaneous leishmaniasis

Isolated, crateriform, ulcerating nodule on right cheek.

236   Cutaneous leishmaniasis

Sharply defined infiltration with central scar formation and peripheral scaling, resembling discoid lupus erythematosus.

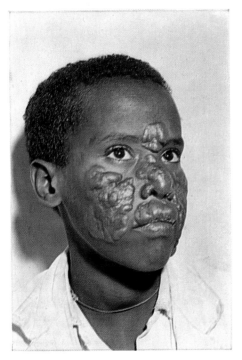

237 Cutaneous leishmaniasis

Nodular-tuberous lesions of the face
with involvement of the lips.

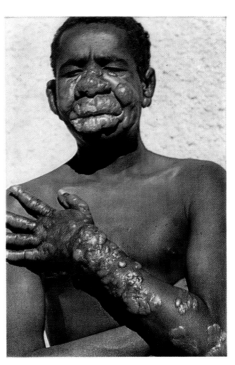

238 Cutaneous leishmaniasis

Multiple nodular infiltrations of the skin
extending to mucous membranes (simulating mucocutaneous leishmaniasis).

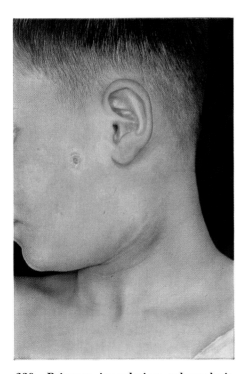

240 B.C.G. inoculation

Simulating primary inoculation tuberculosis. Ulceration of
gluteal inoculation site and perforation of regional lymph
nodes.

239 Primary inoculation tuberculosis

Tuberculous primary complex. Indurated ulcer with prominent lymphadenopathy in a young boy.

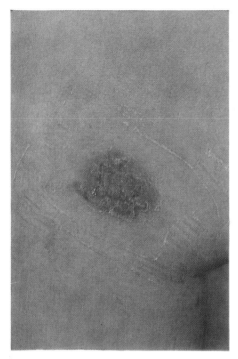

241 Lupus vulgaris
Originating at B.C.G. inoculation site.

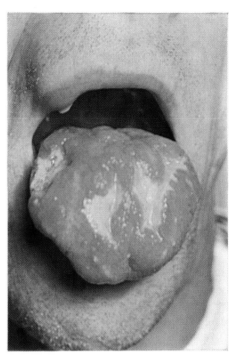

242 Tuberculosis cutis orificialis
Rapidly ulcerating indolent lesions of
the tongue.

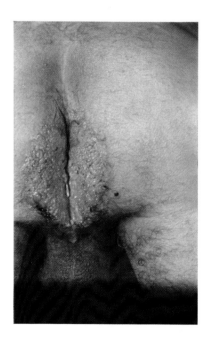

243 Tuberculosis cutis orificialis
Perianal ulcerating and papillomatous tuberculous lesions associated with pulmonary
and visceral tuberculosis.

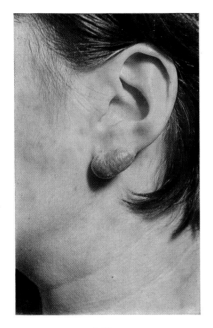

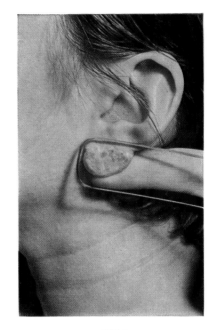

244   245

244 and 245   Lupus vulgaris
Diascopic examination reveals multiple, small, nodular infiltrations
of apple jelly color.

246   Lupus vulgaris
Small, erythematous, infiltrated patch of the
left cheek.

247   Lupus vulgaris
Erythema, infiltration, and scaling of the nose.

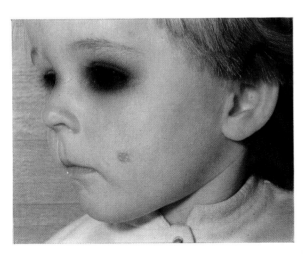

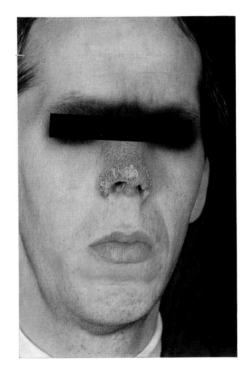

246   247

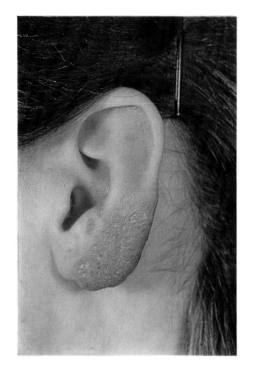

248 Lupus vulgaris
Of the left ear lobe.

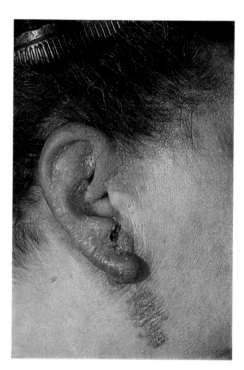

249 Lupus vulgaris
Of the ear, spreading to periauricular
skin.

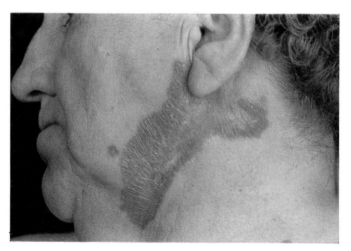

250 Lupus vulgaris
Sharply marginated, erythematous, scaling plaque.

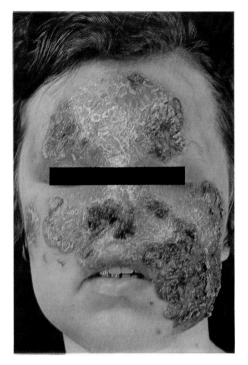

251

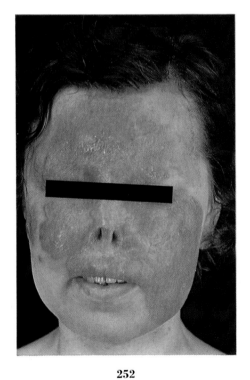

252

253

251, 252 and **253   Lupus vulgaris**

Widespread lesions of the face with heavy crusts and ulceration before, during,
and after INH therapy. Typical "worn-off" appearance of nose.

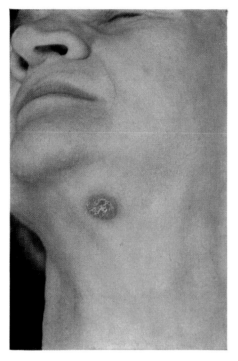

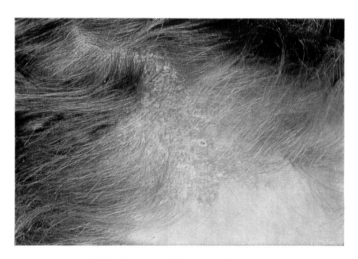

254 Lupus vulgaris

Originating from a deep tuberculous lymph node.

255 Lupus vulgaris of the scalp

Often causing permanent hair loss.

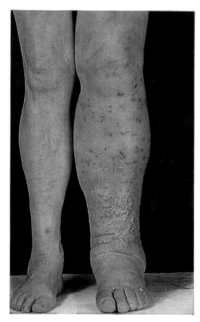

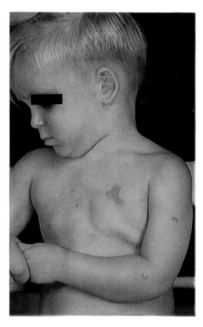

256 Lupus vulgaris

Superimposed on elephantiasis of the left leg.

257 Lupus vulgaris

Multiple lesions in exanthematous distribution.

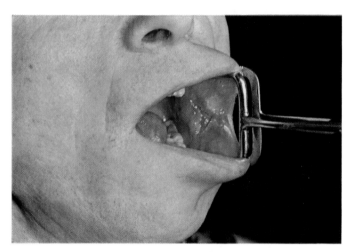

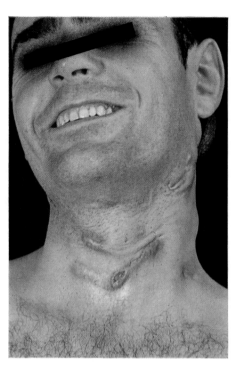

258 Lupus vulgaris
Extensive ulcerative lesions of the buccal mucosa.

259 Scrofuloderma
Ulcerating lymph nodes with fistulous openings healing with hypertrophic scars.

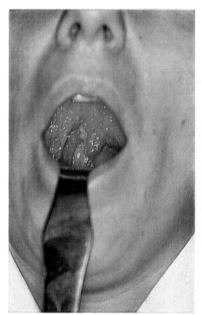

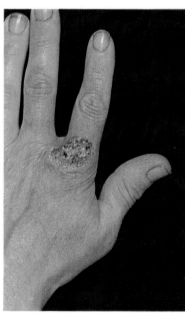

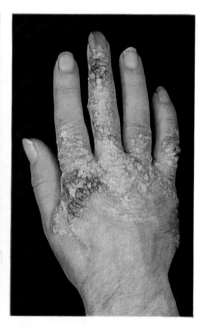

260 Lupus vulgaris
Of the oral mucosa, involving the soft palate and uvula.

261 Tuberculosis verrucosa cutis
Crusted verrucous plaque on the dorsum of the hand.

262 Tuberculosis verrucosa cutis
Widespread, vegetative, verrucous lesions with slight purulent discharge.

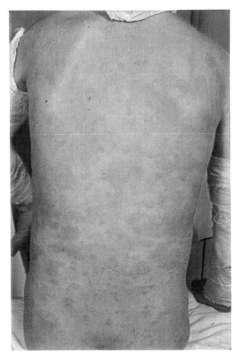

263   Lichen scrofulosorum
Disseminated patches of firm lichenoid papules.

264   Papulonecrotic tuberculid. Most lesions have healed with typical, varioliform, depressed scars.

265   Papulonecrotic tuberculid.
Indolent, reddish-brown, necrotic papules and hyperpigmented depressed scars.

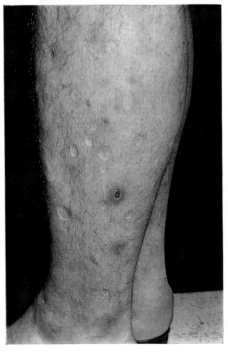

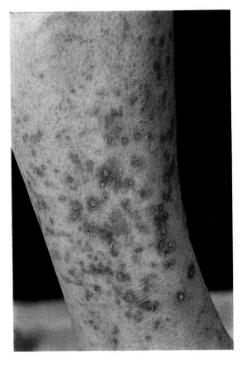

264   **265**

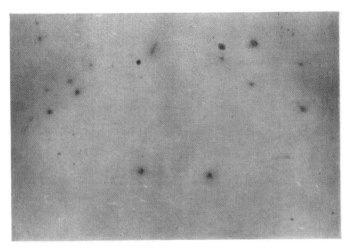

266 Papulonecrotic tuberculid

Early stage with reddish-purplish papules, some with necrotic centers.

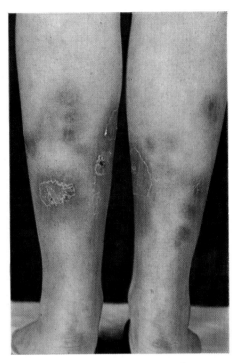

267 Erythema induratum (BAZIN)

Nodular discolored lesions of the calves with ulceration and scarring.

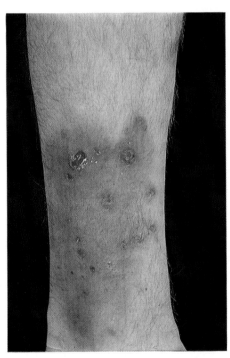

268 Erythema induratum (BAZIN)

Induration, hyperpigmentation, ulcers, and healed lesions on the lower leg.

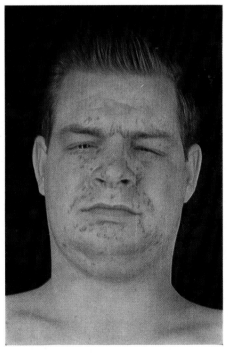

269 Lupus miliaris disseminatus faciei

Symmetrical, small, soft, reddish-brown nodules of the face.

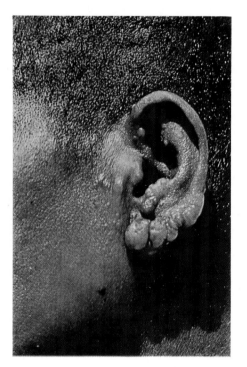

270 Lepromatous leprosy
Nodular infiltration of the ear lobe, a
commonly involved area.

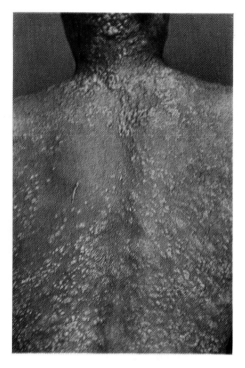

271 Lepromatous leprosy
Extensive papular exanthem.

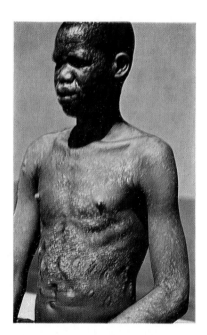

272 Lepromatous leprosy
Widespread nodular infiltration
of the skin.

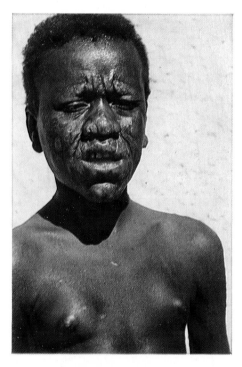

273 Lepromatous leprosy
Nodular infiltration of the face, partial loss of
the eyebrows and eyelashes; gynecomastia due
to endocrine changes following lepromatous
infiltration of the testes.

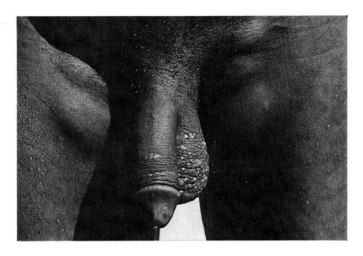

274   Lepromatous leprosy
Papular and nodular lesions of the scrotum with massive
regional lymphadenopathy.

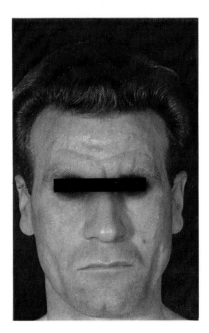

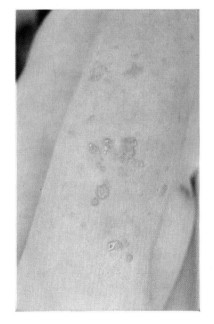

275   **276**

275 and **276   Lepromatous leprosy**
Of the face and arms.

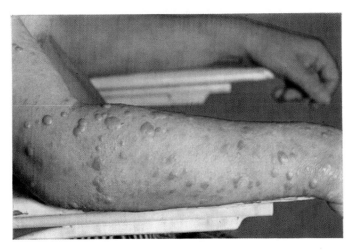

277 Lepromatous leprosy
Nodular infiltrates (lepromas) of the arm.

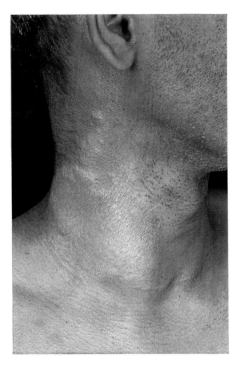

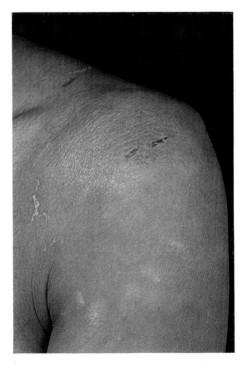

278   **279**

278 and **279** **Tuberculoid leprosy**
Asymmetrical, slightly raised, anesthetic, hypopigmented erythematosquamous
lesions on the neck and shoulder.

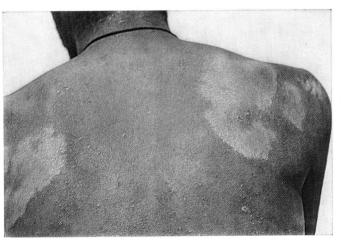

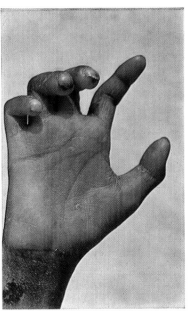

280   Tuberculoid leprosy
Sharply outlined, slightly raised, anesthetic, depigmented lesions with central clearing.

281   Tuberculoid leprosy
Ulnar clawhand due to paralysis of ulnar nerve.

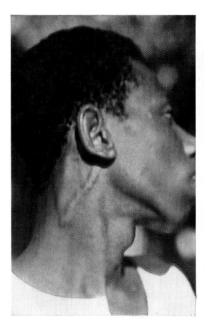

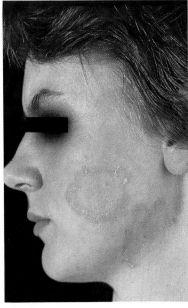

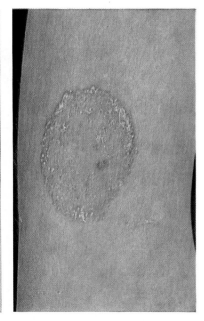

282   Tuberculoid leprosy
Fusiform thickening of a nerve (N. auricularis magnus), a typical finding in tuberculoid leprosy.

283   Tinea corporis
Annular and gyrate lesions with slightly elevated vesicular and scaling border. Spontaneous clearing of the central portion of the lesions.

284   Tinea corporis
Oval lesion with erythema, vesiculation, and scaling, particularly of the border of the lesion.

7*

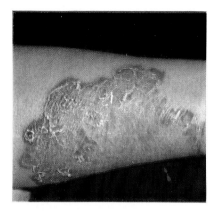

285 Tinea corporis

Tinea of several years' duration, clinically suggestive of lupus vulgaris. The demonstration of fungi, a favorable response to griseofulvin, and the presence of pruritus differentiate these two diseases.

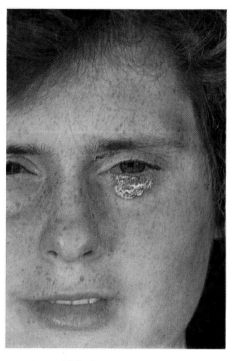

286 Tinea corporis

Unusual localization on the lower lid.

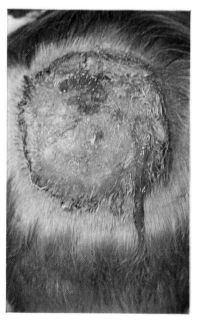

287

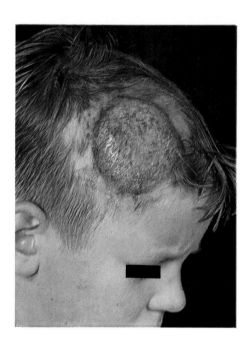

288

287 and 288 Kerion of the scalp

Well defined, soft, succulent lesions with partial hair loss and purulent discharge.

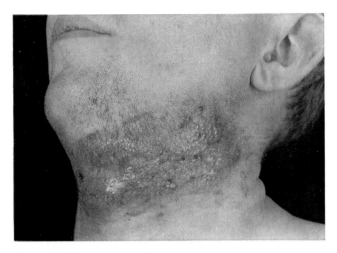

289 Tinea barbae (sycosis barbae)
Elevated, dome-shaped, soft, purulent, nodular lesions
with irregular surface.

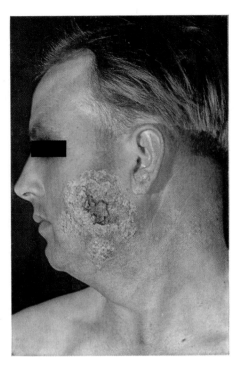

290 Tinea barbae (sycosis barbae)
With scaling and crust formation.

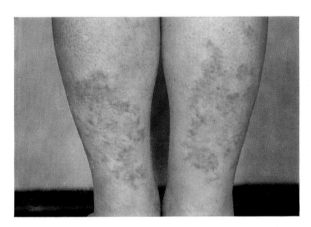

291 Follicular dermatophytosis
Deep pruritic nodules of the lower legs.

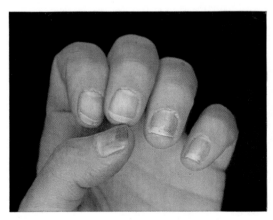

292

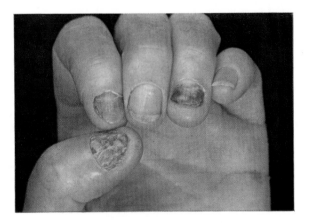

293

292 and 293 Tinea unguium (onychomycosis)
Dirty yellowish-gray discoloration and brittleness of nail plate, usually beginning at the lateral
or distal portion of the nail.

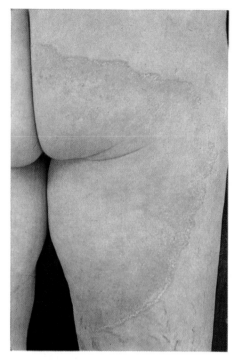

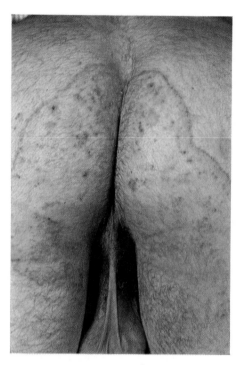

294 Tinea cruris et inguinalis

Sharply marginated large lesion with raised border and slight scaling.

295 Tinea cruris et inguinalis

Sharply defined, raised, erythemato-vesicular border.

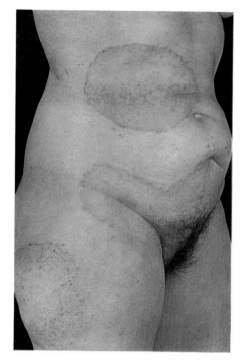

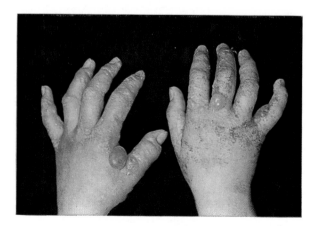

296 Tinea corporis

Multiple large circinate and oval lesions.

297 Tinea manus, dyshidrotic variety

With many vesicles and large bullae.

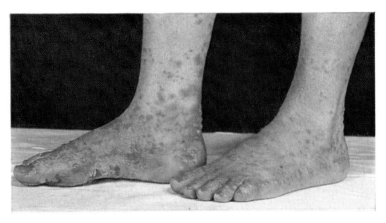

298 Tinea pedis, dyshidrotic variety
With small, red, maculopapular and vesicular lesions.

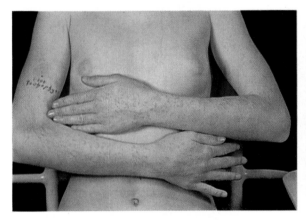

299 Dermatophytid of the hands and arms
Positive trichophytin reaction.

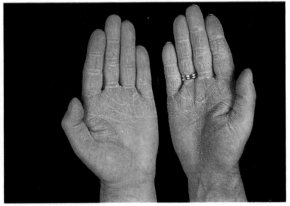

300 Tinea manus, squamous hyperkeratotic variety
Often due to trichophyton rubrum.

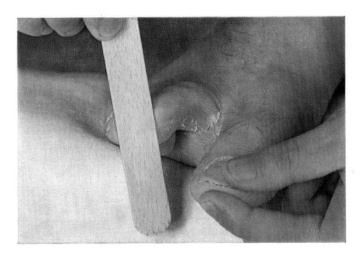

301 Tinea pedis, intertriginous variety
With erythema, scaling, maceration, and fissures of interdigital area.

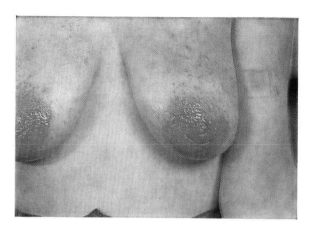

302   Eczematized tinea of the breasts
Rare localization. Positive trichophytin reaction on the upper arm.

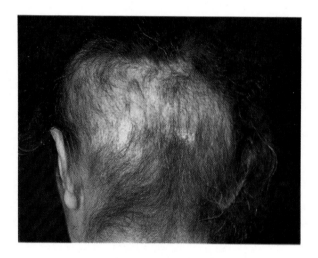

303   Favus
In an oriental patient. Lamelliform scaling, often healing
with alopecia and depressed scars.

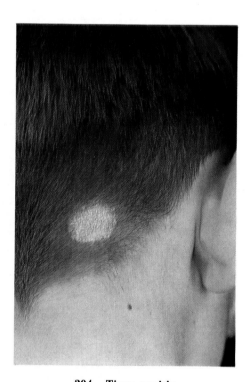

304   Tinea capitis
Sharply marginated round patches with
whitish pityriasiform scaling and short
broken-off hairs.

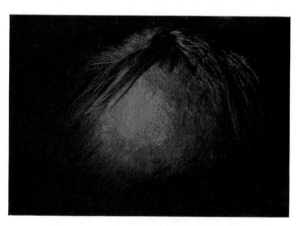

305   Tinea capitis
Fluorescence under Wood's light.

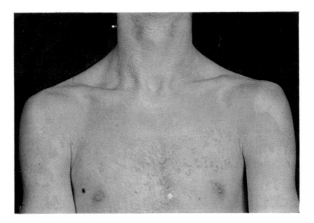

306   Tinea versicolor
Yellowish-brown, confluent lesions with pityriasiform scaling.

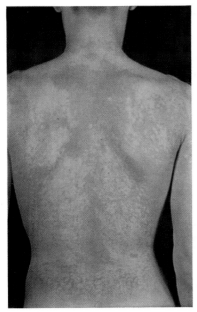

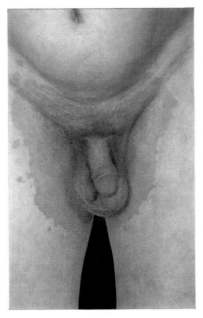

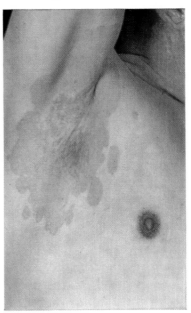

307   Tinea versicolor alba
Acting as an ultraviolet filter, the scales and fungi prevent tanning of the affected areas.

308

309

306 and 307   Erythrasma
Extensive inguinal and axillary involvement in the same patient. The lesions show coral red fluorescence under Wood's light.

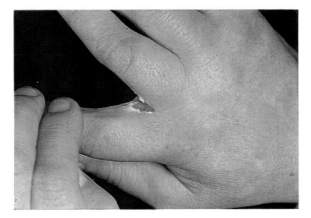

310   Interdigital moniliasis (erosio interdigitalis blastomycetica). Moist erosion with whitish macerated skin.

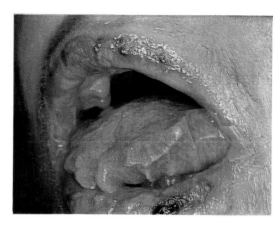

311

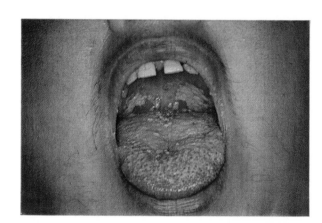

311 and **312**   **Thrush (moniliasis of the oral cavity)**
Erythema, edema, and whitish coating
of mucous membranes.

312

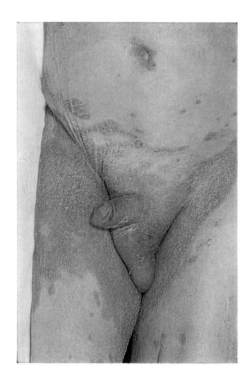

313   **Moniliasis of the skin.** Well defined, erythematosquamous areas with small, pustular,
satellite lesions in a patient with diabetes mellitus.

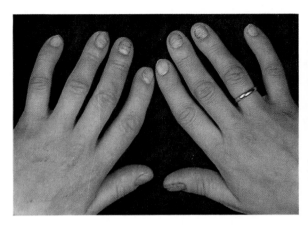

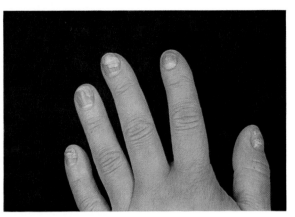

314 Chronic monilial paronychia
Erythema and tender swelling of nail folds with
secondary changes of the nail plate.

315 Moniliasis of the nails (candida albicans)
Resembling onychomycosis due to
dermatophytes.

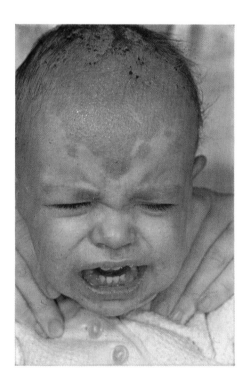

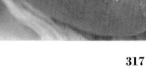

316

317

316 and **317** **Granulomatous moniliasis**
Involving skin, nails, mucous membranes, and intestine.

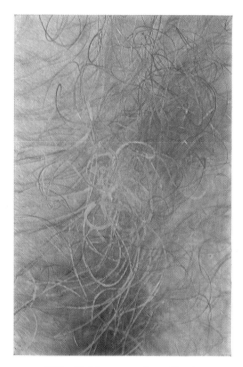

318 Trichomycosis axillaris

The axillary hairs are sheathed in a yellowish, rough, and sticky coating consisting of pigment-forming micrococci and Nocardia tenuis. This disorder is more common in hyperhidrotic patients.

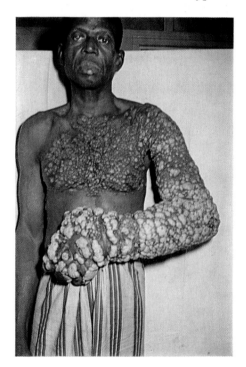

319 Chromoblastomycosis

Brownish and whitish verrucous and papillomatous lesions on the left arm and trunk.

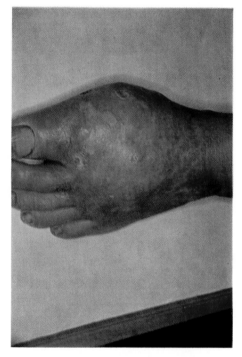

320 Mycetoma (Madura foot)

Nodular, granulomatous, draining process, eventually leading to deformity and destruction of the foot.

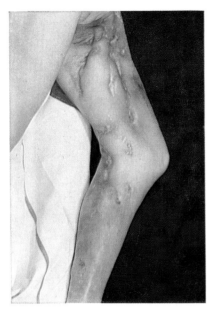

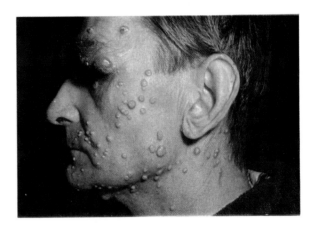

321 Primary actinomycosis of the skin

Hard tender infiltration with sinus tracts and purulent discharge.

322 Mollusca contagiosa

Discrete, globular, umbilicated, nontender nodules of varying size. Lesion on upper lid might be confused with a furuncle or a tumor.

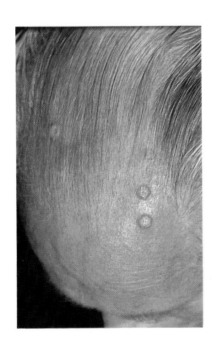

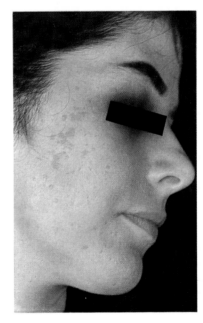

323 Mollusca contagiosa of the scalp

Patient was referred with a diagnosis of "multiple sebaceous gland nevi."

324 Verrucae planae juveniles

Discrete and coalescent reddish-brown flat polygonal papules.

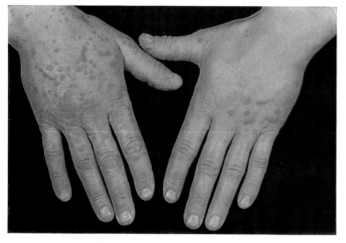

325   Verrucae planae juveniles
Unusually widespread involvement of
the dorsa of the hands with Koebner
phenomenon of the right hand.

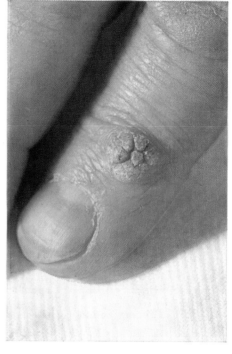

326   Verruca vulgaris
Typical hard, raised, verrucous tumor
with irregular horny surface.

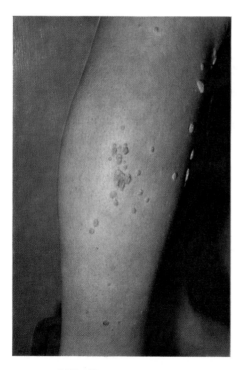

327   Verrucae vulgares
A primary wart is surrounded by smaller
lesions disseminated by scratching
(autoinoculation).

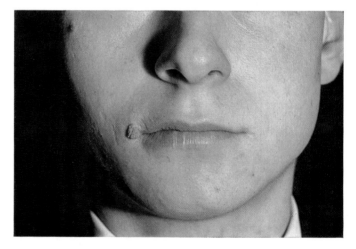

328   Verruca vulgaris
Hard verrucous tumor on the right
corner of the mouth.

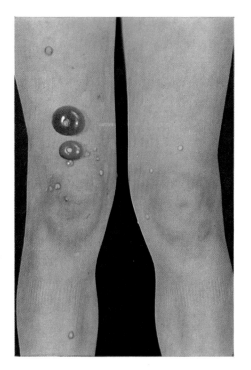

329 Verrucae vulgares

Multiple warts on both legs. Two hemorrhagic blisters induced by liquid nitrogen treatment.

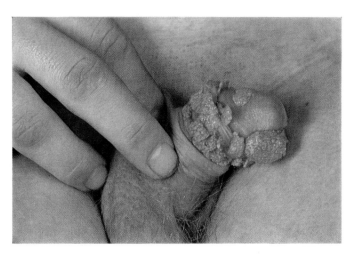

330 Condylomata acuminata

Typical cauliflower-like, soft, moist, reddish papillary tumors on the prepuce and in the coronary sulcus, over the frenulum and on the glans penis.

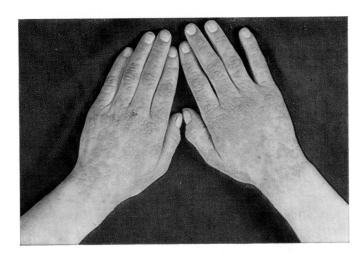

331 Epidermodysplasia verruciformis (LEWANDOWSKY-LUTZ)

Numerous discrete and confluent, raised and flat verrucous lesions on the dorsa of the hands.

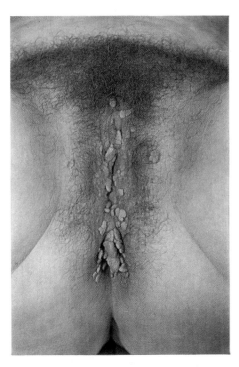

332 Condylomata acuminata

Large lesions on the labia majora and minora and in the perianal area.

112

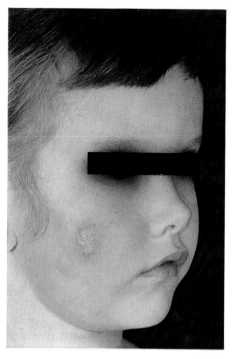

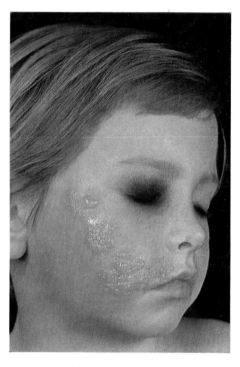

333 Herpes simplex
Multiple eroded vesicles recurrent in identical location.

334 Herpes simplex
Recurrent eruption with typical grouped vesicles on erythematous base.

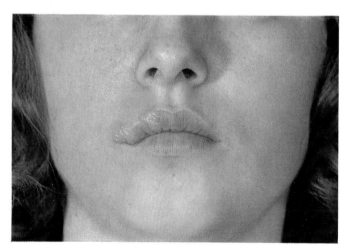

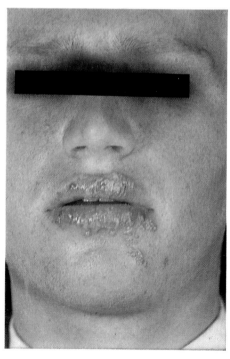

335 Herpes simplex (febrilis)
Small grouped vesicles on erythematous and edematous base.

336 Herpes simplex
Elicited by excessive sun irradiation (herpes solaris).

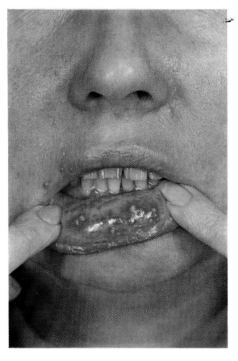

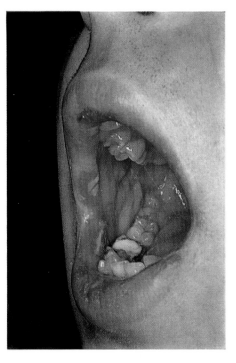

337   Herpes simplex

Some vesicles are still intact; others have become eroded, giving rise to small ulcers.

338   Herpetic gingivostomatitis

Aphthous primary herpes simplex infection of the oral mucosa.

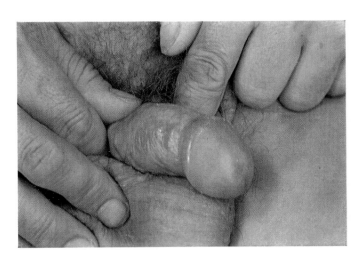

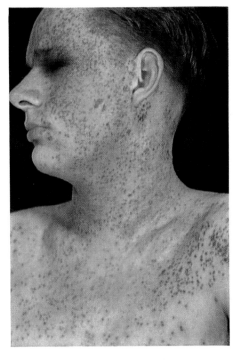

339   Herpes progenitalis

In this location, herpes simplex lesions erode rapidly; consequently, only flat erosions are seen.

340   Eczema herpeticum

Numerous umbilicated, partially eroded, herpes simplex lesions spreading centrifugally from the face; superimposed on atopic dermatitis.

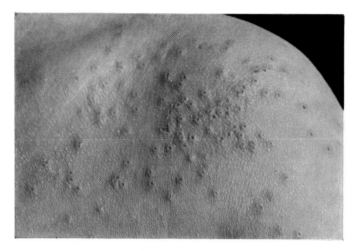

341   Eczema herpeticum
On the shoulder of an atopic patient. Characteristic discrete
umbilicated herpes simplex lesions

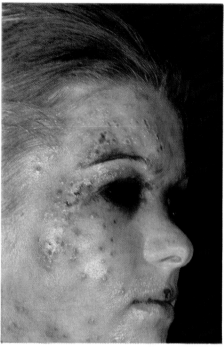

342   Eczema herpeticum
Typical umbilicated vesicles on erythematous, edematous base involving
the face.

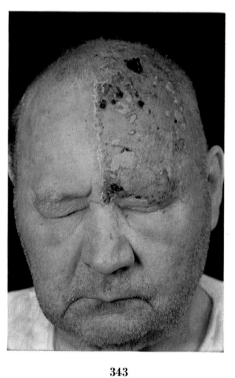

343   **344**

343 and 344   Gangrenous zoster
Following the ophthalmic nerve, involving skin of the forehead, part of the scalp,
the upper eyelid, and the upper portion of the nose.

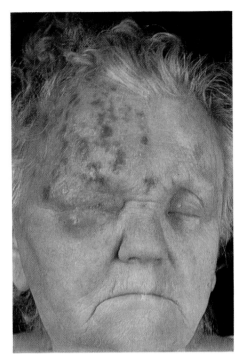

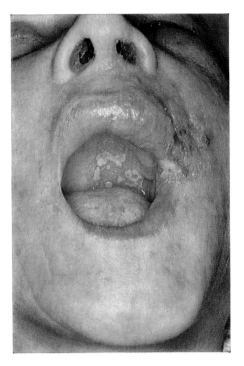

345   Ophthalmic zoster

Strictly confined to the area of the ophthalmic nerve. Hemorrhagic vesicles
with necrotic base.

346   Zoster

Grouped vesicles following the distribution of the maxillary nerve, involving
skin of the left cheek, the upper lip,
and the oral and nasal mucosa. Skin and
mucous membrane lesions are often
preceded by severe toothache.

347 and 348   Zoster

Typical herpetic, grouped, hemorrhagic vesicles
and pustules extending from C 6 to T 2.

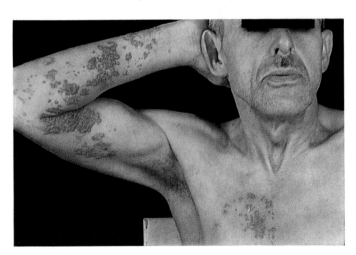

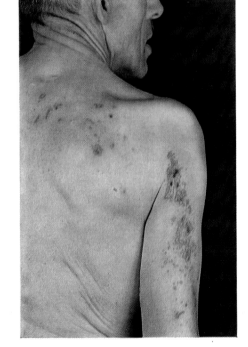

347

348

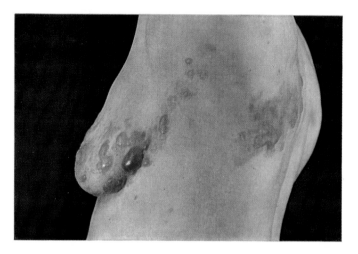

349 Zoster

Large bullae and vesicles in a patient with chronic lymphatic
leukemia (at level of T 4 and T 5).

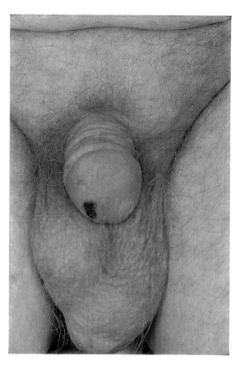

350 Zoster

Necrotizing vesicular lesions of glans
penis (S 3).

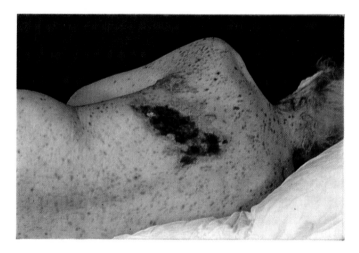

351 Generalized zoster

Associated with chronic lymphatic leukemia.
Deep necroses in the thoracic segments 4 and 5.

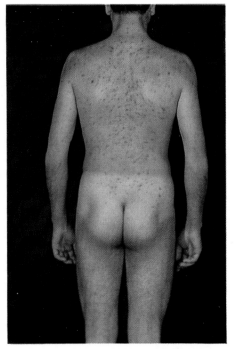 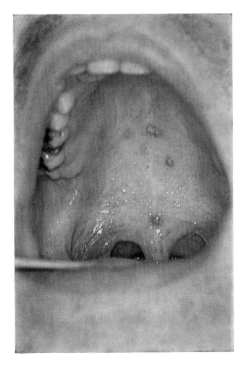

352 353

352 and 353 Varicella in an adult patient

Exanthematous lesions in different stages of development (macules, papules, vesicles, pustules, and crusted lesions present simultaneously). Enanthema of oral mucosa with vesicular lesions of the hard palate.

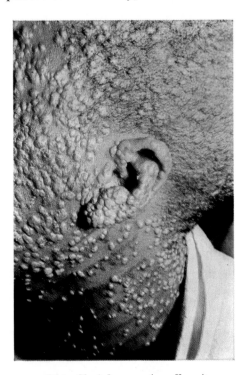 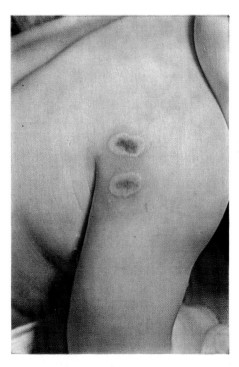

354 Variola vera (smallpox)

Generalized eruption with typical umbilicated pustules on an erythematous base associated with severe systemic symptoms. In contrast to varicella, all lesions are in same stage of development.

355 Smallpox vaccination

Between the seventh and ninth day after vaccination, the initial vesicle develops into a large necrotic pustule. The surrounding area assumes an erysipeloid appearance, and the regional lymph nodes become enlarged.

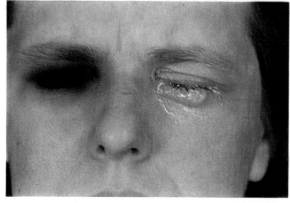

356   Inoculation vaccinia

On the eyelid of a woman with practically no residual immunity.

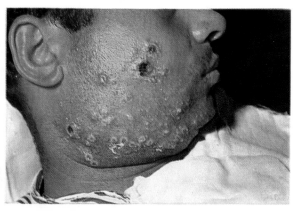

357   Inoculation vaccinia

Umbilicated and necrotic pustules in a patient who had never been vaccinated.

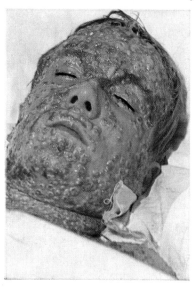

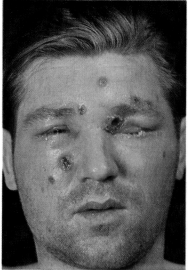

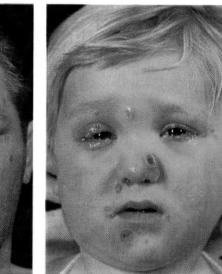

358   Eczema vaccinatum

Typical coalescing umbilicated pustules, superimposed on atopic dermatitis.

359   **359 and 360   Cowpox**   **360**

In a farmhand and his daughter. Umbilicated blisters and pustules on an edematous base, especially pronounced in the orbital region.

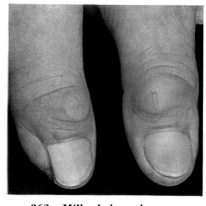

361   Milker's nodule

Infection with paravaccinia virus.

362   Milker's hyperkeratoses

Callus-like, hard, horny lesions due to milking technique. No viral disease.

Sarcoidosis and related diseases

Sarcoidosis (Besnier-Boeck-Schaumann)

Besnier (1889) described lupus pernio; Boeck (1899), multiple lesions of benign sarcoidosis of the skin. In 1904, Kreibich reported several cases of lupus pernio with multiple lesions on other parts of the integument, and fusiform swelling of the fingers with cystic radiolucent defects of the phalanges. The term, *ostitis fibrosa multiplex cystica* was first used by Jüngling (1919) to describe these osseous changes. Schaumann was one of the first to recognize the characteristic pulmonary changes which resemble miliary tuberculosis.

Histologically, sarcoidosis is characterized by a tuberculoid reaction with epithelioid cells. In the United States, a large percentage of the patients are Negroes. It is a disease of adults and is more common in females. The *superficial disseminated form* of Besnier-Boeck-Schaumann disease, also known as benign miliary lupoid, presents pinhead- to pea-sized maculopapular or lichenoid isolated skin lesions of reddish-brown to livid coloring. Diascopy reveals yellowish-brownish punctate infiltrations. Occasionally, the nodules coalesce into serpiginous or annular lesions.

The *nodular form* of the disease is characterized by separate, brownish to bluish-red, indurated nodules which could be as large as a walnut. Subcutaneous nodules of the lower legs are known as the Darier-Roussy type of sarcoidosis. When the nodules show a more purple coloring resembling frostbite (pernio), they are referred to as lupus pernio. The systemic nature of sarcoidosis is emphasized by such findings as hilar lymphadenopathy, miliary pulmonary infiltrations, ostitis multiplex cystica and fusiform swelling of the phalanges, Heerfordt syndrome (uveoparotic fever) and Mikulicz syndrome (involvement of lacrimal and salivary glands), and involvement of lymph nodes, liver, or other internal organs. Total serum protein is usually elevated (increase in gamma globulins). Hypercalcemia is a frequent finding. Some authors consider sarcoidosis an atypical form of tuberculosis; the tuberculin skin test is negative. Others believe the disease to be a syndrome that may have a variety of causes.

Melkersson-Rosenthal syndrome

This syndrome is characterized by recurring edema of the lips and upper face, facial paralysis or paresis, and scrotal tongue. Systemic symptoms are absent. Tuberculosis and allergic processes have been discussed as etiologic factors.

Cheilitis granulomatosa (Miescher)

Typical features are progressive swelling of the lips and macrocheilia, which may become permanent; some authors consider this disease a monosymptomatic form of Melkersson-Rosenthal syndrome.

Granuloma annulare (Radcliffe-Crocker)

This disease has a predilection for the extensor surfaces of the fingers, the dorsa of the hands, the external ear, and the dorsa of the feet; occasionally, disseminated eruptions are seen. The lesions are small, nontender, sharply defined, deep-seated, firm papules or nodules which are skin-colored, whitish or slightly erythematous. They spread centrifugally, forming annular configurations with normal-appearing centers. The disease is easily diagnosed and has a favorable prognosis. It is common in children and young adults; rarely, tuberculosis may be found to be an etiologic factor. In some cases, a rheumatic hyperergic reaction may be present.

120

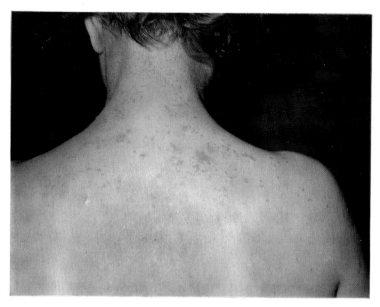

363   Sarcoidosis (benign miliary lupoid)
Superficial disseminated variety. Reddish maculopapular lesions of the back.

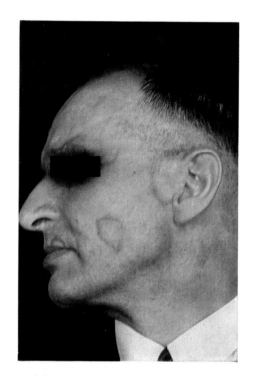

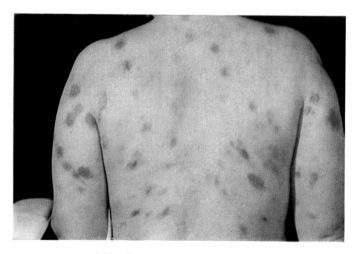

365   Sarcoidosis, nodular type
Bluish-red, firm nodules in the face, on the trunk, and on the extremities. Yellowish-brownish punctate infiltrations are seen under diascopic examination.

364   Sarcoidosis, annular variety

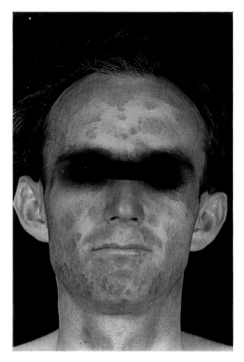

366 Sarcoidosis
Brownish-red, coalescent, infiltrated patches of the face and neck.

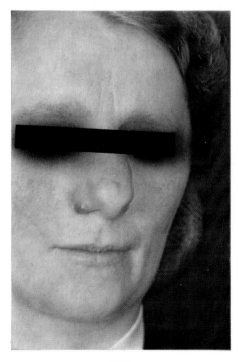

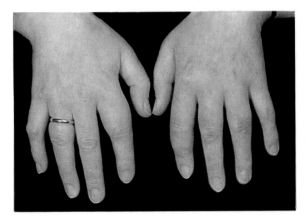

367

368

367 and 368 Sarcoidosis
Bluish indurated nodule of the nose (lupus pernio) and fusiform swelling of the fingers
due to ostitis multiplex cystica.

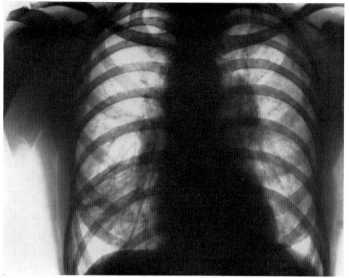

369 Sarcoidosis

Radiograph of case illustrated in figure 367. Lungs show hilar lymphadenopathy and miliary pulmonary infiltrations.

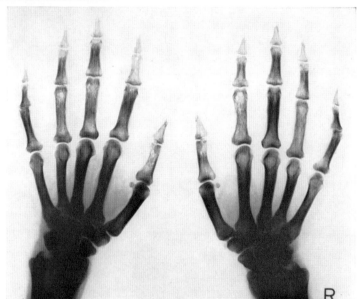

370 Sarcoidosis

Typical cystic, radiolucent defects of phalanges (ostitis multiplex cystica KREIBICH-JÜNGLING). Same patient as shown in figure 368.

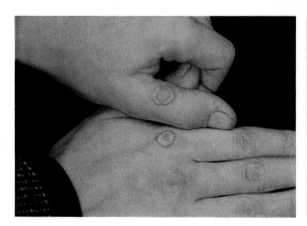

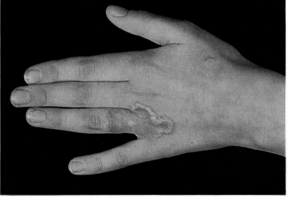

371 Granuloma annulare

Hard, annular lesions with raised border.

372 Granuloma annulare

Firm, gyrate lesion with central healing and peripheral growth.

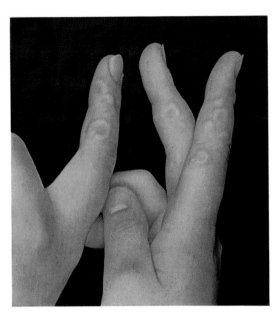

373   Granuloma annulare

Solitary, annular, and arciform indurated skin lesions.

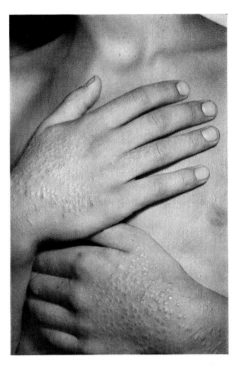

374   Disseminated granuloma annulare

Multiple small, raised, firm lesions on the dorsa of the hands and fingers.

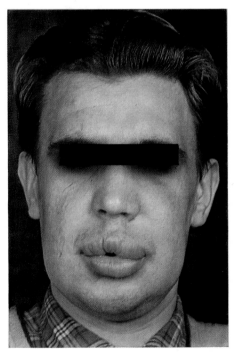

375

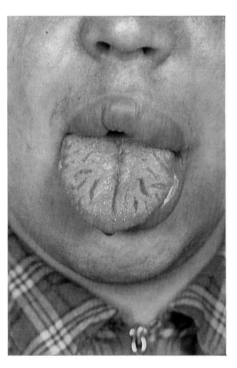

376

375 and 376   Melkersson-Rosenthal syndrome

Recurrent edema of the lips, left facial paresis, and scrotal tongue.

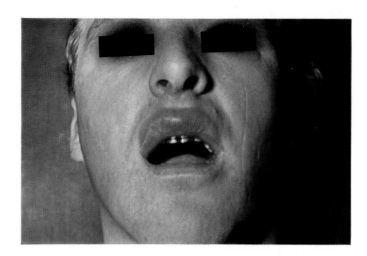

377 Cheilitis granulomatosa (Miescher)
Progressive inflammatory edema of the upper lip.

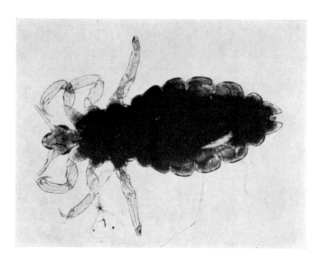

378 Body louse (pediculus corporis)
The body louse is longer than the head and
pubic louse.

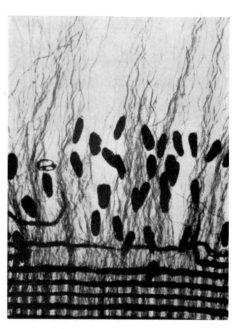

379 Nits of body louse
Usually found in seams of clothing.

Zoonotic dermatoses

Pediculosis capitis

Infestation with the head louse (Pediculus capitis), which is smaller and more slender than the body louse (Pediculus corporis) is usually due to poor scalp hygiene. Its eggs (nits) are glued in long rows to the scalp hair, usually beginning at the temporal aspects; frequently, however, the entire scalp is involved. The infestation causes itching, and the resulting scratching leads to secondary changes of the scalp with oozing and impetiginization. The hair may become matted. Whereas a severe case of pediculosis is easily diagnosed, it may be difficult to detect live lice on a fairly well groomed scalp. A useful diagnostic point is the fact that dandruff is easily removed from the hair, while nits are firmly attached.

Pediculosis corporis

The mobile body louse is found on skin areas covered by clothing. Its eggs (nits), shiny, transparent, ovoid, conspicuous structures, often of the same color as their background, are deposited on fibers and seams of clothing. Newly hatched lice are so small that they can be visualized only with a lens. Once one member of a household is affected, the infestation usually spreads rapidly to other members. Since the parasites also invade furniture and blankets, disinfection of every room and all clothing is indicated.

Pediculosis pubis

The pubic louse (Phthirus pubis), of greater width than length, has strong claw-like extremities which firmly grip the infested hair. The parasite is flat, pale gray, and readily detected when in motion, but easily mistaken for a small crust when immobile. The infestation usually begins in the pubic area, then spreads along the trunk to the axillary hair. Occasionally pubic lice may be found in the ciliary and superciliary hair of adults, where they may cause conjunctivitis, and on the scalps of children. A secretion transmitted by their bites produces pigmented steel gray-blue spots, so-called "tâches bleues" (maculae caeruleae). The nits, deposited on the hair, are provided with a coverlet which remains open after the lice have hatched. Excoriations are usually absent because patients suffering from pediculosis pubis tend to "rub" rather than scratch.

Scabies

Scabies is caused by a mite, Acarus or Sarcoptes scabiei. The female deposits her eggs in burrows deep in the horny layer of the skin. In addition to eggs, these tunnels contain fecal and other matter. The larvae hatch after $2\frac{1}{2}$ to 3 days and reach sexual maturity within 2 to 3 weeks. The males stay on the surface of the skin, usually in skin folds, and die after copulation. Sites of predilection are the soft parts of the skin, particularly the interdigital spaces of the fingers; in young children, the palms and soles also may be involved. In adult males, the external genitals are not infrequently affected, and in females the nipple area may be involved. The burrows may be straight, angular, or curved, and have a slightly raised, vesicular, erythematous area at their terminal point. Subsequently, papules and vesicles covered with crusts develop on the wrists, in the antecubital areas, and in the anterior axillary folds, less frequently on the legs, back, neck, and face. Various degrees of excoriations are seen, depending on the severity of the pruritus. In chronic cases, impetiginization and eczematization may occur. The diagnosis is established by demonstration of the burrows and of the parasites in potassium hydroxide preparations.

Animal mites that may be transferred to man temporarily are Dermanyssus avium, Acarus equi, Acarus cani, Acarus cati, and mites living in foodstuffs, cereals (grain itch), and straw, such as Pediculoides ventricosus. Their bite induces papules and similar reactions, thus producing a scabies-like clinical picture. However, these mites do not dig burrows in the skin, but live on the skin surface for short periods of time; they may be visualized with a lens.

Tick bites

Pruritic nodules, papules, or urticarial reactions can be caused by tick bites. Ticks occur in woody and scrubby territory and penetrate into the skin of man and animals upon contact. Engorged with blood, the parasite becomes a bean-sized, spherical or pear-shaped, bluish-black structure. A common method of removing the ticks is by touching it with oil, glycerin, gasoline, or a lighted cigarette; usually, however, the head is torn off during this manipulation and causes local inflammation of the skin. Ticks are also important as vectors of infectious diseases.

Pulicosis (Flea bites)

The human flea (Pulex irritans), a wingless insect 2 to 4 mm. in length, has become quite rare. Through its bite, a hyperemia-producing and coagulation-inhibiting secretion is injected into the tissue; the human skin reacts to this irritant by forming wheals and papules with characteristic tiny hemorrhagic puncta in the center. Vesicular reactions, secondary infections, and even purpura pulicosa have been encountered.

Culiosis (Mosquito bites)

Flies are a common pest, especially near stagnant waters. Their bites produce wheals with central puncta, or — especially in children — bullous reactions. *Papular urticaria* (strophulus infantum) is in most cases due to hypersensitivity to flea, bedbug, and other insect bites. It is a common disease of children between 2 and 7 years of age and occurs during the summer months. It consists of numerous papules, urticarial lesions, and excoriations, particularly in exposed skin areas.

Creeping eruption (Larva migrans)

The typical migratory, tortuous, threadlike, urticarial lesions correspond to the burrowing of different larvae in tropical climates. The most common types are caused by various larvae of Ancylostoma (helminthiasis) or botflies (myiasis).

Filariasis

Pathologic changes produced by various filaria in the human organism are lymphangitis, lymphadenopathy, and obstruction of the lymph vessels resulting in elephantiasis of the genitals and lower extremities (Wuchereria bancrofti), cutaneous nodules (Onchocerca volvulus), ulcerations and inflammatory skin changes on the feet and lower legs (Dracunculus medinensis), and transient allergic reaction of the skin (Loa loa). The filarial parasites are nematodes found in the tropics; they are transmitted by various species of Culex, Cinopheles, and Aedes, and produce microfilaria which require suitable hosts for their development.

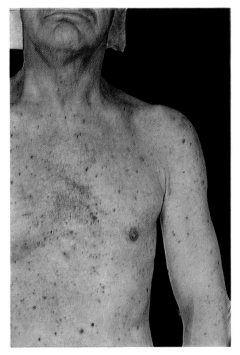

380 Pediculosis corporis (body lice)

Excoriations with secondary infection,
superficial scarring, and hyperpigmentation (vagabond's disease).

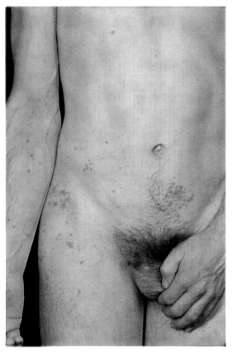

381   Flea bites

Wheals with central puncta and petechiae. Characteristically, the lesions
occur in groups.

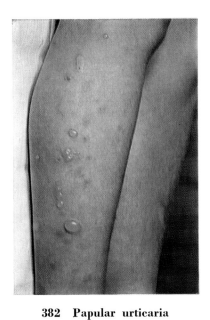

**382   Papular urticaria
(strophulus)**

Papular, urticarial, and bullous reaction due to mosquito
bites.

383   Creeping eruption

Starting with a punctate erythematous lesion, a linear urticarial
eruption 2 to 3 cm. in length developed within 30 minutes and subsided after a few hours.

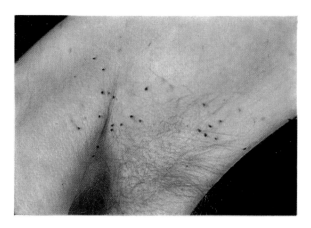

384 Ticks (Ixodes ricinus)

Many small ticks in the axillary region causing pruritic papules
and urticarial lesions.

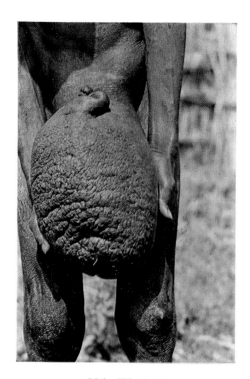

385 Filariasis

Unusually large elephantiasis of the
scrotum.

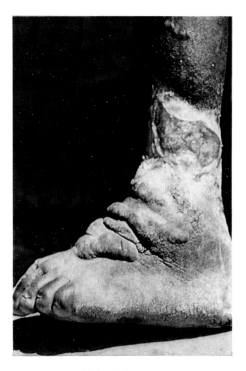

386 Filariasis

Elephantiasis of lower leg with secondary pyoderma and ulceration.

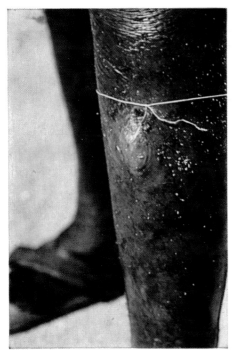

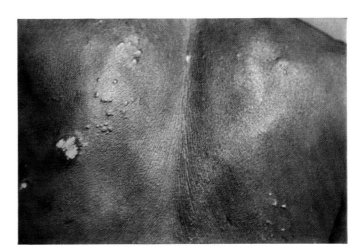

387 Dracunculus medinensis

The parasite extracted from the leg is fastened with a string tied around the leg. The extracted, somewhat dehydrated portion of the parasite is seen pointing toward the right.

388 Onchocercosis

Typical subcutaneous nodules of varying size, containing the adult filaria. Secondary ulceration of some areas.

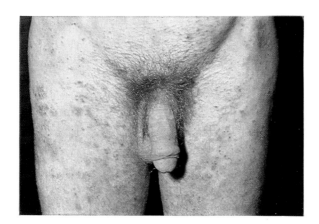

389 Scabies

Inflamed burrows in widespread papulovesicular lesions of the thighs with many excoriations and punctate hemorrhagic crusts.

Hereditary Cutaneous Disorders

This group comprises skin diseases widely differing in their symptomatology, but united by the fact that they are inheritable.

Ichthyosiform and Keratotic Genodermatoses

Ichthyosis vulgaris (Fish skin disease)

This disease is inherited as a simple dominant of variable expressivity. The symmetrical, large, quadrilateral, plate-like, centrally adherent scales with loose edges are usually absent at birth; they develop during the first years of life. Areas of principal involvement are the trunk and the extensor aspects of the extremities. In addition, punctate follicular hyperkeratotic papules (keratosis pilaris) are frequently observed on the lateral surfaces of the extremities.

In *ichthyosis simplex (xeroderma)*, the face, the antecubital areas, palms and soles are usually not involved. In *ichthyosis nitida*, the scales are more conspicuous, shiny and translucent. *Ichthyosis nigricans* is characterized by dirty gray to black scaling. Circumscribed papular, verrucous, spinous, and plate-like horny scales may be seen in severe forms of ichthyosis. The term *ichthyosis hystrix* is sometimes used for large verrucous epithelial nevi; they are not related to ichthyosis.

Ichthyosis congenita

This disorder is transmitted as a recessive characteristic. In contrast to ichthyosis vulgaris, the hyperkeratotic changes are usually present at birth. Three clinical variants of the same basic condition, with different severity of clinical symptoms, can be differentiated. The *gravis type* with hyperkeratoses present in utero, results in stillbirth or early death of the newborn (*harlequin fetus:* erythema, hyperkeratoses, deep fissures, ectropion). The *larvate type* shows various transitional forms of keratotic skin changes. In contrast to ichthyosis vulgaris, the flexor surfaces of the large joints are always involved. The *tardive type*, usually less severe, presents hyperkeratotic changes during the first 2 years of life.

Congenital ichthyosiform erythroderma (Brocq)

This rare genodermatosis is associated with erythroderma and lamellated scaling; it is usually transmitted as a recessive. According to Kogoj, the disease is a variant of the larvate type of ichthyosis congenita. Bullous forms have been reported.

Other authors consider the disease an inflammatory variant of ichthyosis vulgaris which is differentiated clinically by involvement of the flexor surfaces. In adults, the inflammatory component is less pronounced.

Erythrokeratoderma

Erythro- et keratoderma figurata variabilis (Mendes da Costa type) is one of several forms of erythrokeratoderma having a high familial incidence and a dominant pattern of inheritance. Reddish-yellow, sharply defined, partially coalescing skin lesions covered with dry grayish scales and presenting a hyperkeratotic border may appear soon after birth or during early adult life. The keratotic changes may become unusually extensive.

Pachyonychia congenita
(Jadassohn-Lewandowsky)
(Keratosis multiformis idiopathica)
(Siemens)

Changes of the nails and multiple anomalies of keratinization of the skin and mucous membranes are usually present at birth. The nail plates are thickened and firmly attached. Keratotic follicular lesions (keratosis pilaris) are seen on the extensor surfaces of the extremities. Occasionally, hyperhidrosis, abnormalities of hair, teeth, and bone development, bulla formation, and mental deficiency are observed. The pattern of inheritance is unknown. Familial incidence with strong sex limitation to males has been reported.

Keratoma palmare et plantare hereditarium
(Keratosis palmaris et plantaris)
(Unna-Thost)

The affected areas, usually the palms and soles, are covered with a yellowish horny layer of even thickness. The disease is inherited as a dominant, it usually manifests itself during the first 2 years of life. A 1 cm. red border separates the keratoma from the surrounding normal skin.

Mal de Meleda
(Keratoma palmare et plantare transgrediens)
(Siemens)

This is a diffuse symmetrical keratoderma, usually beginning on the palms and soles. It progressively involves the dorsa of fingers, hands, toes, forearms and lower legs. The disease is transmitted as a recessive characteristic. Greither described a dominant form under the name of *keratosis extremitatum hereditaria progrediens.*

Keratoma palmare et plantare dissipatum hereditarium (Brauer)

The punctate, cone-shaped, horny lesions seen in shallow depressions of the skin on the palms and soles usually occur at the beginning of the third decade of life. The horny plugs may be shed, leaving pit-like scars. The disease is inherited as a dominant condition.

Arsenical keratoses also present as punctate palmar lesions.

Keratosis palmo-plantaris mutilans
(Pardo-Costello and Mestre, Vohwinkel)

This palmoplantar keratosis spreads to fingers and toes where it produces spontaneous amputation by linear constriction (pseudo-Ainhum).

Keratosis follicularis (Darier)

The primary lesions are small firm papules developing in follicular orifices or on normal skin. Each lesion is covered by a yellowish-brown crust; the base is sometimes erythematous. The papules have a tendency to coalesce and develop into papillomatous, dirty and greasy patches. Areas of predilection are the chest, back, sacral area, scalp, face, dorsa of the hands, and body folds. Decomposition of the horny masses results in exudation, irrita-

tion, and an unpleasant odor, especially in creases and folds of the skin where maceration develops easily. Irregularly shaped papillomatous growths may develop underneath the keratotic masses. "Formes frustes" are characterized by lesions on the back of the hands reminiscent of flat warts. The oral mucous membranes may show flat nodules and irregular papillary lesions.

The disease may have its onset in the first year of life, usually later. In all cases, even in mild forms, characteristic interruptions of the dermatoglyphics of the palms can be observed.

Inheritance of the disorder is of the autosomal irregular dominant type.

Keratosis pilaris
(Lichen pilaris, keratosis suprafollicularis)

This is a very common abnormality, presenting as discrete conical hyperkeratoses of the follicular orifices. The corneous plugs often enclose fine lanugo hairs. The lesions are seen predominantly in adolescents, on the extensor aspects of the extremities and in the gluteal area. Patients with ichthyosis vulgaris often show similar changes. A variant of keratosis pilaris in the eyebrow region is *ulerythema ophryogenes,* with horny follicular papules surrounded by a persistent erythema. These lesions may leave atrophy and scars.

Hyperkeratosis follicularis et parafollicularis in cutem penetrans (Kyrle)

Discrete, deep, horny plugs, sometimes coalescing into polycyclic configurations, penetrate into the cutis. When the follicular hyperkeratoses are removed, a small depression can be seen. This rare disease occurs on the thighs, axillae, chest, and abdomen.

Elastosis perforans serpiginosa (Miescher)
(Keratosis follicularis serpiginosa) (Lutz)

Small papules form linear lesions with a verrucous keratotic surface in serpiginous or disseminated arrangement, most frequently on the neck, but also in other skin regions. Most patients are teenagers or young adults. The disease is self-limited. Association with defects of other organ systems has been described.

Other Genodermatoses

Adenoma sebaceum (PRINGLE)
(Epiloia) (Tuberous sclerosis)

This disease, inherited as a dominant condition, is quite variable in its symptomatology. It usually manifests itself in the first decade but becomes more prominent during pubescence. The most common symptom combination occurs in the form of a triad consisting of mental deficiency, epilepsy, and various skin tumors. Among these are organic sebaceous gland nevi (the term "adenoma sebaceum" is a misnomer) in the form of multiple, rounded, firm, skin-colored or red papules or nodules in the central portion of the face, often associated with telangiectases, peri- and subungual fibromas on the toes and fingers (KOENEN's tumors), verrucous pigmented nevi on the trunk, and pinhead sized papillomatous nodules on the oral mucosa, especially the gingiva. Tumors of the retina (phacomas), brain tumors (gliomas), and atypical mixed tumors of internal organs are also seen. The disease is probably related to neurofibromatosis.

Neurofibromatosis
(VON RECKLINGHAUSEN)

This systemic disease, transmitted as an irregular dominant condition, originates from immature nerve cells or SCHWANN cells. Typical symptoms of neurofibromatosis are numerous oval, brownish-yellow "café au lait" spots, with a relatively smooth border, on the trunk and extremities (more than six are considered diagnostic); pigmented nevi or freckles; vascular nevi; soft rounded or pendulous skin-colored neurofibromas; neurinomas; elephantiasic tissue accumulations (dermatolysis); tumors of the spinal nerves and the spinal canal; intracranial tumors; neurofibromas of internal organs; skeletal abnormalities; retinal tumors (phacomas); hypertrichosis of the sacral region; endocrine disturbances; mental deficiency; and psychic alterations. Abortive oligosymptomatic forms are seen occasionally.

Hereditary hemorrhagic telangiectasia
(RENDU-OSLER-WEBER)

The essential symptoms of this familial disease are numerous sharply circumscribed red macules and papules with telangiectases on lips, face, nasal and oral mucous membranes, and internal organs; also epistaxis and secondary anemia due to internal hemorrhages. An autosomal dominant gene governs this abnormality.

Familial acroosteolysis (GIACCAI)

Indolent ulcers of the soles, with bone sequestration following febrile attacks, trophic changes of the skin, and deformities of the feet are suggestive of osteolysis of the phalanges and the metatarsal bones. This familial disorder, which is easily demonstrable roentgenologically, is controlled by a dominant gene.

Pseudoxanthoma elasticum (DARIER)

This anomaly is most commonly seen in female adults as asymptomatic yellowish to orange-colored papules in linear distribution or leathery plaques, particularly on neck, axillae, face, and groin. Histologically, the changes are limited to the elastic fibers (elastorrhexis). In addition to the skin, elastic changes occur in the fundus of the eye (angioid streaks) leading to impaired vision (GRÖNBLAD-STRANDBERG syndrome), in the cardiovascular system (angina pectoris, hypertension, intermittent claudication, gastrointestinal hemorrhages). The disorder is ingerited primarily as an autosomal recessive, rarely as an autosomal dominant characteristic.

Knuckle pads (GARROD) (Heloderma)

True "knuckle pads" are plaque-like fibromatous thickenings on the extensor surfaces of the proximal interphalangeal joints of the fingers. Inflammatory changes are absent. Cases of familial incidence and combination with DUPUYTREN's contracture have been reported. Etiologic factors are of a genetic and non-mechanical nature. *Pseudo-"knuckle pads,"* on the other hand, are callus formations entirely due to mechanical pressure.

Cutis hyperelastica
(EHLERS-DANLOS)

This rare dystrophic anomaly is characterized by cutaneous hyperextensibility, extreme fragility of the skin and of the blood vessels resulting in hematomas and atrophic changes in areas of frequent trauma, and hyperflexibility of the joints. It is inherited as a dominant trait, but may occur in the absence of demonstrable genetic factors. Blue sclerae, epicanthal folds, and aortic aneurysms are common in this condition.

Congenital anhidrotic ectodermal defect

The characteristic symptoms of this usually recessive entity, which is sex-linked to males and only rarely inherited as a dominant trait, are absence or paucity of sweat glands with marked intolerance to heat, hypoplasia of sebaceous glands, dental abnormalities, atrophy of the nasal mucosa (often with typical saddle nose), impairment of salivary and lacrimal secretion, corneal dystrophy, nail changes, and — frequently — hypotrichosis.

Peutz-Jeghers *syndrome, xeroderma pigmentosum, hydroa vacciniforme, familial idiopathic hypercholesteremic xanthomatosis, gout,* and Hartnup *syndrome* are other genodermatoses which are discussed elsewhere.

Bullous Genodermatoses

Epidermolysis bullosa simplex

In this abnormality, which is transmitted as a dominant mendelian trait and has a higher incidence in the male sex, minor mechanical trauma induces bullae on exposed areas of the body, particularly on the feet, hands, elbows, and knees. The lesions heal without scarring.

Epidermolysis bullosa dystrophica

Inherited as a recessive or dominant trait, this disorder is characterized by bulla formation following even the slightest degree of traumatization. Other important features are scarring, keloids, milia, dystrophic nails or anonychia, erosions and leukokeratosis of the mucous membranes, hyperkeratosis of palms and soles (hyperplastic type of Touraine), skeletal anomalies, impairment of dentition (polydysplastic type of Touraine), and psychological alteration.

Familial benign chronic pemphigus
(Hailey and Hailey)

This disease is transmitted by a single dominant gene. In young adults, rapidly eroding vesicles appear on the nape and lateral aspects of the neck, the axillae, and the genital area. Coalescence of the lesions results in eczematoid, macerated, crusted lesions, which show a tendency to heal spontaneously from the center. Remissions and recurrences alternate.

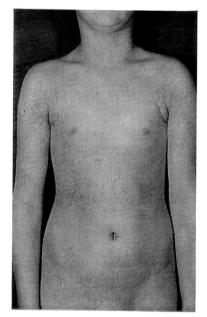

390 Ichthyosis vulgaris

Symmetrical, firmly attached, grayish-white to dirty gray plate-like scales. Characteristically, the antecubital areas are not affected.

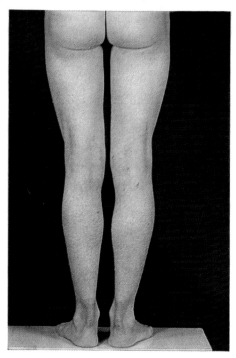

391 Ichthyosis vulgaris

Symmetrical involvement of both legs with the exception of the popliteal areas.

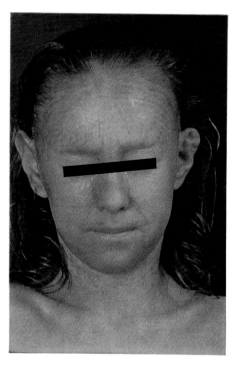

392 Ichthyosis congenita, larvate type

Dry, parchment-like, hyperkeratotic skin present since birth. The flexor aspects of the large joints are also involved.

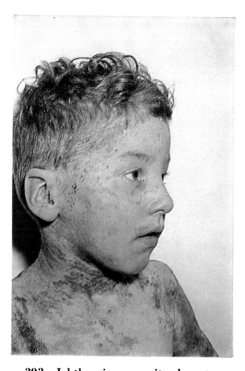

393 Ichthyosis congenita, larvate type

Massive and widespread, hyperkeratotic, partially verrucous changes of the face and trunk, present since birth.

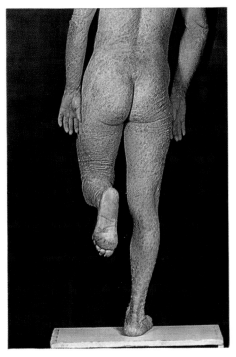

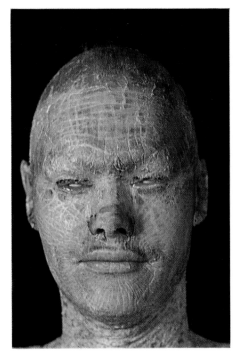

394   **395**

394 and 395   Ichthyosis congenita, larvate type

Parchment-like skin with hyperkeratotic changes resembling fish scales, rigidity of facial expression, hair loss and ectropion. Typically, the popliteal areas, palms, and soles are also affected.

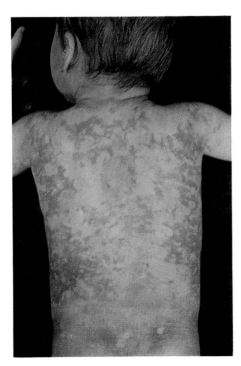

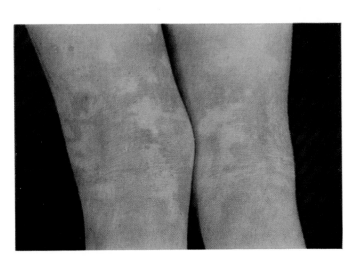

396   **397**

396 and 397   Congenital ichthyosiform erythroderma

Hyperkeratotic areas with erythema and scaling; popliteal areas are also involved.

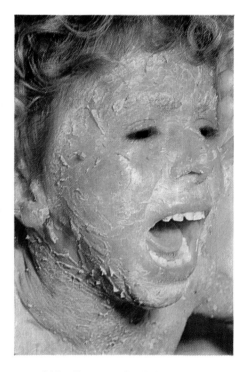

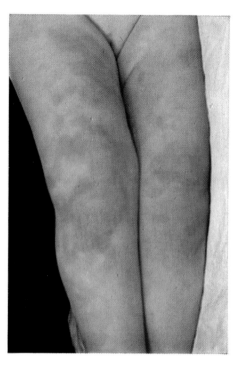

**398 Congenital ichthyosiform
erythroderma**

Marked erythema and massive lamelliform scaling, with involvement of the
flexor aspects of the large joints.

399 Erythrokeratoderma figurata variabilis
(MENDES DA COSTA)

Onset of disease during the fourth month of life. The girl's
father (fig. 399) and grandfather suffered from the same
disease. The 1-year-old girl shows a geographic pattern of
distinct new reddish and older brownish lesions with a
slightly accentuated surface pattern. Hyperkeratoses, which
are pronounced in the father, are not yet visible in the child.

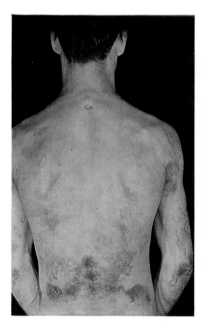

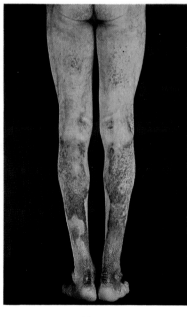

400 and **401**
**Erythrokeratoderma figurata
variabilis** (MENDES DA COSTA)
Sharply defined, erythematous,
scaling lesions with marked dark
hyperkeratoses.

400

401

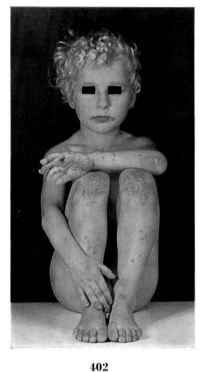

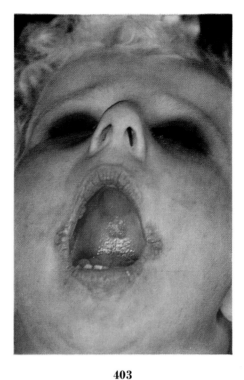

402

403

402 and 403   Congenital pachyonychia (Jadassohn-Lewandowsky)

Firmly attached, thickened, dull, yellowish nail plates with broken distal edges.
Follicular and coalescent hyperkeratotic skin lesions and leukokeratosis of the palate.

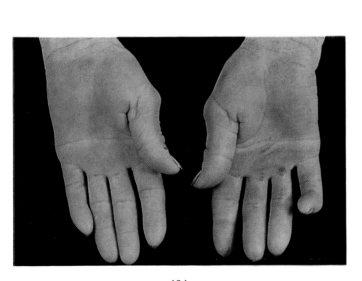

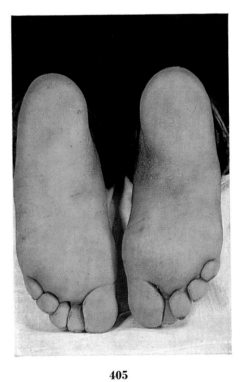

404

405

404 and 405   Keratoma palmare et plantare hereditarium (Unna-Thost)

Keratosis palmaris et plantaris with hard horny masses of even thickness.

138

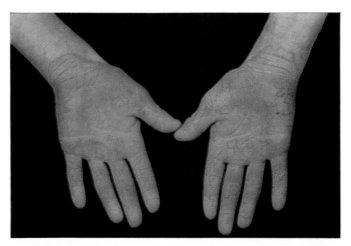

406

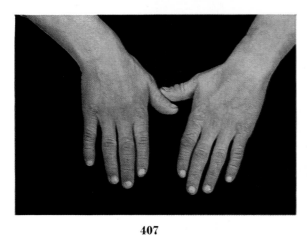

407

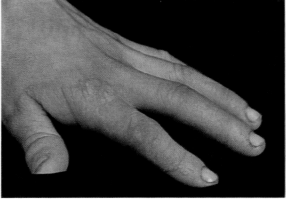

408

406, 407 and **408   Keratosis hereditaria palmo-plantaris diffusa**
Punctate horny lesions and thick hyperkeratotic patches of irregular outline on an erythematous base.

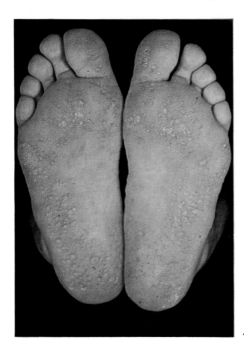

410

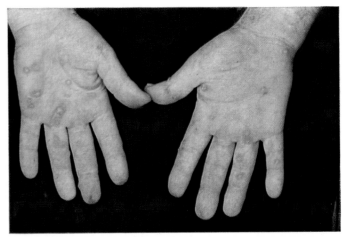

409

409 and **410   Keratoma palmare et plantare dissipatum hereditarium.** Discrete and coalescent, small, hyperkeratotic lesions with erythematous border on the soles and palms.

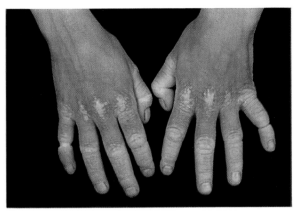
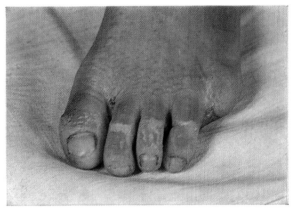

411   **412**

411 and 412   Keratosis palmo-plantaris mutilans
Keratotic lesions of the palms, soles, fingers, and toes causing bandlike constrictions
of the fingers and spontaneous amputation of the fifth toe.

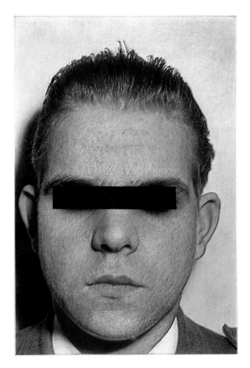

413   Keratosis follicularis (DARIER)
Coalescing yellowish-brown papules with irregular greasy crusts
covering the entire face.

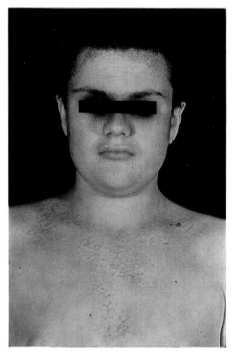

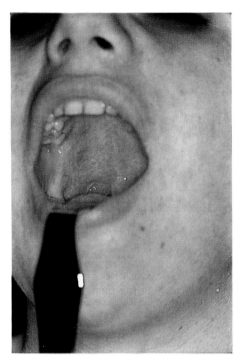

414 Keratosis follicularis (Darier)

The lesions are especially numerous in areas with high sebum production (face, hair line, ears, sternal area).

415 Keratosis follicularis (Darier)

Small flat papules of the palate. Mucosal lesions are not uncommon.

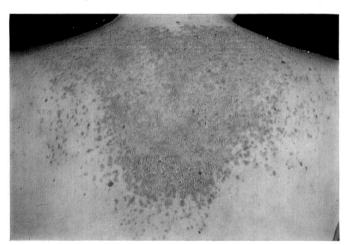

416 Keratosis follicularis (Darier)

Typical involvement of the upper back at the interscapular region. Large hyperkeratotic area with peripheral discrete and coalescent greasy grayish-brown papules.

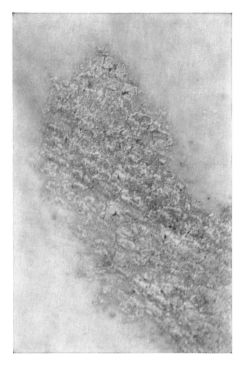

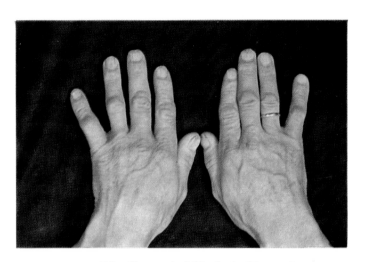

417   Keratosis follicularis (DARIER)
Hyperkeratotic, partially macerated, and scaling greasy yellowish-brown lesions in the right inguinal area.

418   Keratosis follicularis (DARIER)
Small, flat, papular lesions on the dorsa of the hands, easily confused with flat warts.

421   Hyperkeratosis follicularis et parafollicularis in cutem penetrans (KYRLE)
Discrete, hard, deep hyperkeratotic plugs, necrotic lesions, and small scars of the lower leg. ↓

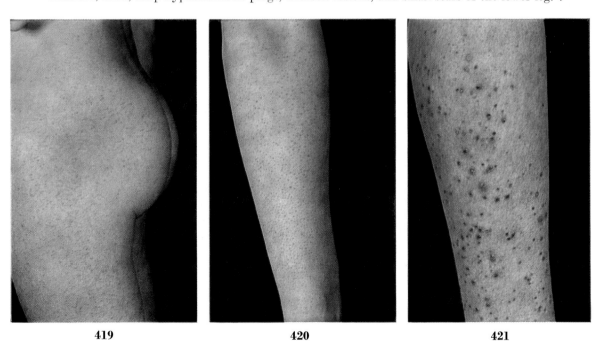

419   420   421

419 and **420   Keratosis pilaris**
Small, discrete, follicular horny plugs with mild erythema on the
gluteal region and extremities.

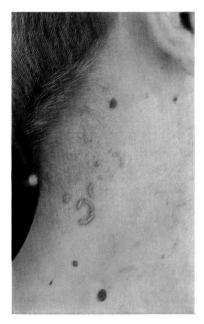
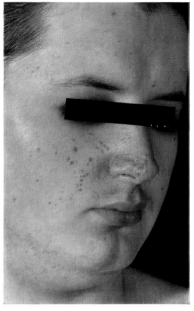

**422 Elastosis perforans serpi-
ginosa** (Miescher)

Linear hyperkeratotic papules in
circinate and serpiginous arrangement on the lateral neck.

423 Adenoma sebaceum
(Pringle)

Small, reddish-yellow, firm nodules surrounded by normal skin
on the nose and cheek.

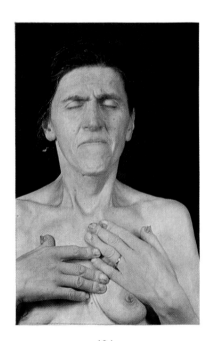
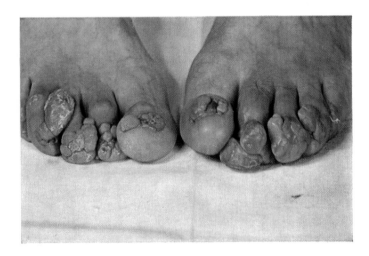

424

425

424 and 425 Adenoma sebaceum (Pringle)

Typical red firm papules of the face and large fibromas (Koenen's periungual tumors)
on the fingers and toes.

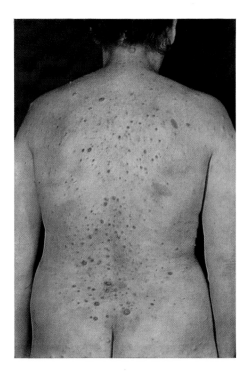

426   Neurofibromatosis (VON RECKLINGHAUSEN)

Numerous soft neurofibromas which may be depressed into the skin in "pushbutton" fashion.
Also, typical "café au lait" spots.

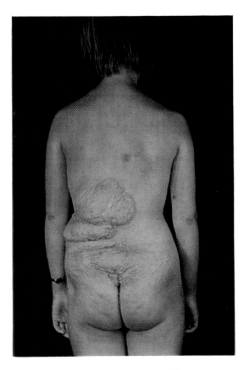

427   Neurofibromatosis (VON RECKLING-
HAUSEN). With large pendulous skin
flaps (dermatolysis).

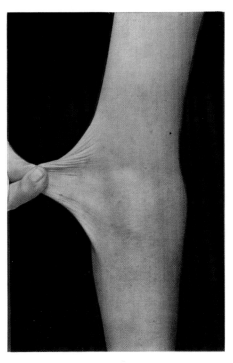

428   Cutis hyperelastica
(EHLERS-DANLOS)

144

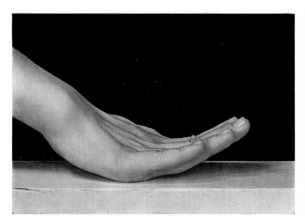

429 Cutis hyperelastica (Ehlers-Danlos)
Hyperflexibility of the joints.

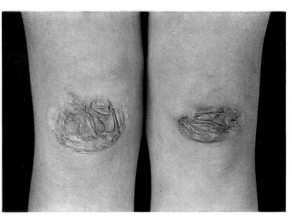

430 Cutis hyperelastica (Ehlers-Danlos)
Increased fragility of the skin resulting
in atrophic scars.

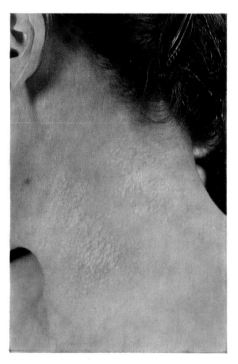

431 Pseudoxanthoma elasticum
Groups of slightly raised, soft yellowish
papules on the lateral aspects of the
neck.

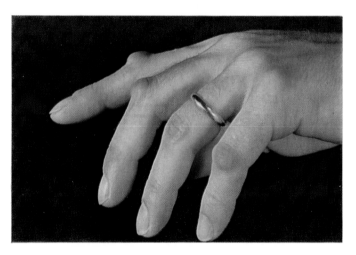

432 Knuckle pads
Fibromatous thickenings on the extensor surfaces of
the proximal interphalangeal joints.

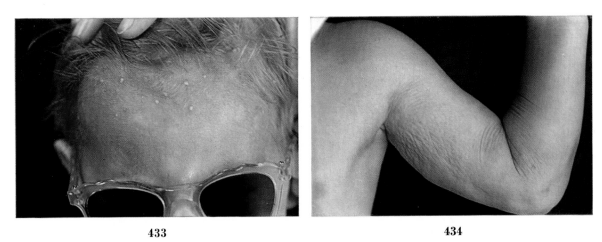

433   434

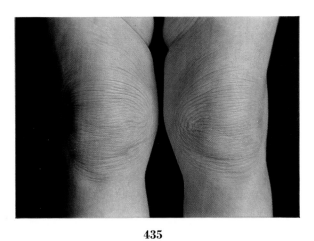

435

433, 434 and 435   Congenital anhidrotic ectodermal defect

Sparse scalp hair of fine texture, milia-like lesions of forehead, scanty eye brows. Skin of extremities is thin, wrinkled, and hairless.

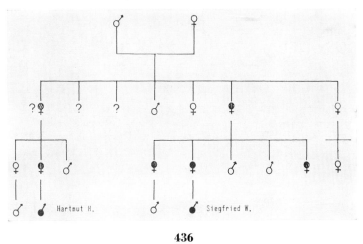

436

436   Congenital anhidrotic ectodermal defect

Family tree showing dominant transmission of the disorder.

146

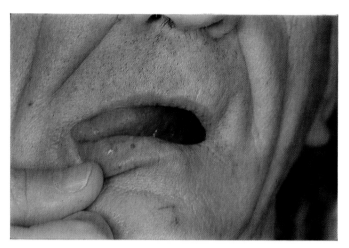

437   Hereditary hemorrhagic telangiectasia
(RENDU-OSLER-WEBER)
Telangiectases and small angiomas on the skin, lips,
oral mucosa, and tongue.

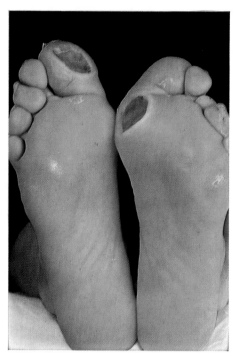

438   Familial acroosteolysis
Indolent ulcers and trophic changes of
the soles and toes.

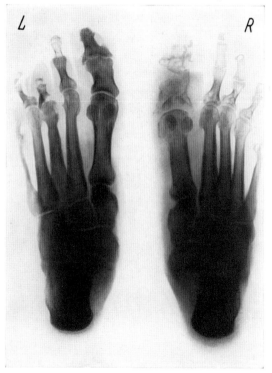

439   Familial acroosteolysis
Osteolytic destruction of bones, particularly of
the right big toe.

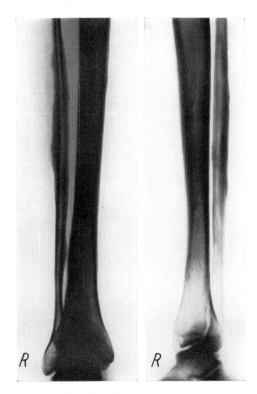

440   Familial acroosteolysis
Irregular thickening of periosteum of the
fibula and tibia.

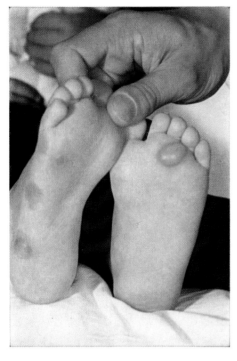

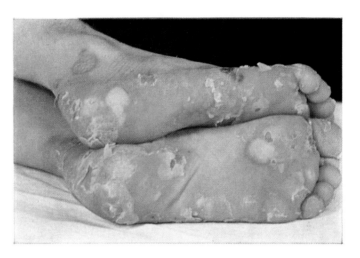

441   Epidermolysis bullosa simplex
Large bullae of the feet; healing without
scarring.

442   Epidermolysis bullosa simplex
Ruptured large bullae and lamelliform
scaling of the soles.

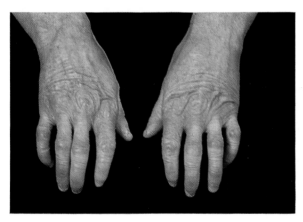

443   **444**

443 and 444   Epidermolysis bullosa dystrophica
Late stage with scarring of the hands, and anonychia of the toes.

10*

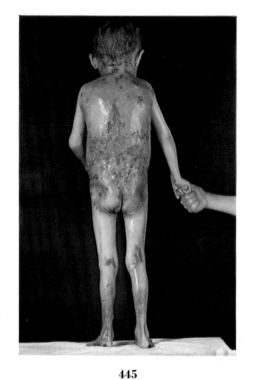

445

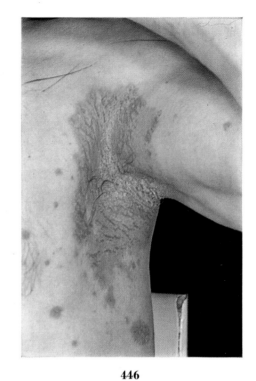

446

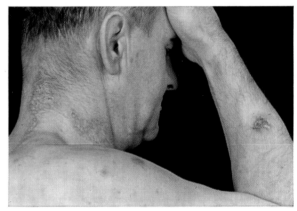

447

448

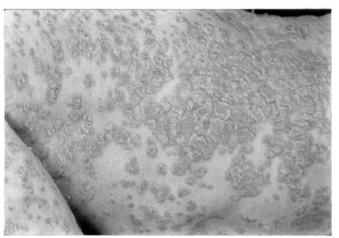

449

**445 Epidermolysis bullosa dystro-
phica (polydysplastic type)**
Severe bullous form with osseous and
dental changes.

**446 Familial benign chronic pem-
phigus** (HAILEY-HAILEY)
Eczematoid, macerated lesions with
small peripheral vesicles.

447, 448 and **449 Familial benign
chronic pemphigus** (HAILEY-HAILEY)
Discrete and coalescent eroded vesicles with crusts, scales, and maceration.

Vesiculobullous Eruptions

Bullae associated with cutaneous diseases of known etiology (bullous syphilid, bullous reactions associated with erysipelas, impetigo, burns, frostbite, insect bites, and allergic reactions of the skin), as well as heritable bullous dermatoses and bullous variants of dermatoses usually characterized by a different morphological pattern, have been described in their respective chapters.

This section is devoted to bullous dermatoses of unknown etiology. They may be divided into three groups: (1) dermatoses with acantholytic blister formation; (2) dermatoses with subepidermal blister formation; and (3) bullous dermatoses associated with pregnancy.

Dermatoses with Acantholytic Blister Formation (Pemphigus Group)

Acantholysis resulting in intraepidermal bullae (CIVATTE, DARIER, TZANCK, LEVER) is the histological criterion of this group. Detached acantholytic cells can be found within the bullae. These cells are rounded and smaller than normal epidermal cells; their nuclei are large; the cytoplasm is condensed and basophilic.

Pemphigus vulgaris

Large blisters may occur in any body region. Occasionally the first lesions appear on the oral mucosa, more rarely on the conjunctivae, without significant systemic impairment. The bullae arise on nonerythematous, clinically normal skin; initially they are tense, later they become flaccid. Firm lateral pressure causes the bullae to spread into the surrounding normal skin (NIKOLSKY's sign). Their clear contents may be hemorrhagic at times. Secondary infection results in cloudy fluid and may produce an inflammatory erythema in the surrounding skin. The bullae rupture readily, producing painful, easily bleeding erosions on skin and mucous membranes, sometimes associated with crust formation. Without massive doses of corticosteroids, this etiologically unclassified disease progressively leads to secondary systemic involvement, cachexia, and death.

Pemphigus foliaceus

In this rare disorder, insignificant flaccid vesicles are followed by moist scaling and flaking of the skin surface without visible bullae. The lesions spread slowly and may involve the entire body surface, resembling a generalized exfoliative dermatitis. This is rarely seen in other types of pemphigus.

Occasionally, pemphigus foliaceus may evolve from pemphigus vulgaris. NIKOLSKY's sign is positive; the mucous membranes are often involved. Malodorous secondary infection of the skin and loss of hair and nails are commonly seen. Impairment of general health is found only in more advanced stages of the disease.

Brazilian pemphigus (Fogo selvagem)

This condition closely resembles pemphigus foliaceus. It occurs as a febrile, endemic, possibly contagious disease in tropical regions of South America.

Pemphigus erythematosus (SENEAR-USHER)

The erythematous, scaling and crusted lesions are clinically suggestive of seborrheic dermatitis (pemphigus seborrhoicus) or lupus erythematosus. They occur mostly in the "butterfly" area of the face. Small bullae also can be seen on the chest and extremities. NIKOLSKY's sign is positive. The disease takes a relatively benign course and may even heal completely. In other cases, recurrent progressive exacerbations eventually lead to the clinical picture of pemphigus foliaceus.

Pemphigus vegetans (NEUMANN)

This rare and often fatal febrile variety of pemphigus shows a preference for the oral or vulvar mucous membranes, and for the intertriginous areas of the axillae, groin, anogenital, and inframammary regions, where it usually forms fetid, purulent, hypertrophic vegetative masses. Erosions develop less frequently than in other type of pemphigus.

150

Dermatoses with Subepidermal Blister Formation

Subepidermal bullae without acantholytic cells can be seen in many skin diseases (e.g., erythema multiforme, porphyria, epidermolysis bullosa). The histological findings are not diagnostic.

Bullous pemphigoid

In this relatively benign and often self-limited disease of elderly people, large and tense, slightly pruritic, nongrouped bullae appear on erythematous, often edematous skin, chiefly on the lateral aspects of the neck, in the axillae, and on the inner aspects of the thighs. Mucous membrane lesions are rare. The disorder can be differentiated from dermatitis herpetiformis by its onset late in life, absence of grouped lesions, and poor response to sulfa-pyridine therapy. Differentiation from pemphigus vulgaris is made histologically (subepidermal bullae).

Chronic course and absence of target lesions exclude erythema multiforme. Drug eruptions must be ruled out. Bullous pemphigoid has a more favorable prognosis than pemphigus vulgaris; the general health is usually not impaired, except in the aged.

Dermatitis herpetiformis (Duhring)

Recurrent polymorphous eruptions, accompanied by intense itching or burning and eosinophilia of the peripheral bood and blister fluid, are characteristic of dermatitis herpetiformis. Herpetiform grouping, symmetrical arrangement, and characteristic appearance of the lesions are distinctive features. Grouped vesicles arise on an erythematous or urticarial base, usually on the extremities and the trunk, in a symmetrical pattern. In other cases, the lesions may be small, indurated papules or crusted vesicles. Gyrate, erythematous, sometimes urticarial patches are often seen initially.

The mucous membranes may be involved. Hyperpigmented areas are late sequelae indicative of preceding active lesions.

The disease is more common in male than in female patients and may occur at any age; usually it appears in middle adult life. Repeated outbreaks are the rule but spontaneous remissions can be expected in many patients. In elderly persons, Duhring's disease may be a manifestation of internal cancer.

Bullous and Pustular Dermatoses Associated with Pregnancy

Herpes gestationis (Milton)

This is a rare papular or vesicular eruption of unknown etiology. It is probably a variant of dermatitis herpetiformis affecting women during pregnancy. In some instances, Rh incompatibility has been demonstrated. The disease usually manifests itself during the first three months of gestation and disappears soon after delivery. Rarely, it may appear postpartum and persist for several weeks.

Impetigo herpetiformis (Hebra, Kaposi)

This exceedingly rare disease predominantly affects pregnant women, usually during the last trimester, but may also occur following thyroid operations, or even in male patients. In most cases, grouped pustules on an erythematous base, often arranged in rings, particularly involve intertriginous areas. Differentiation from psoriasis pustulosa is extremely difficult; possibly, impetigo herpetiformis during pregnancy is merely a pustular form of psoriasis. Some cases seem to be identical with dermatitis herpetiformis. Other findings suggest an endocrinological pathogenesis of the disease, particularly the presence of severe systemic symptoms and the fatal outcome of some cases. Maceration, secondary infection, nephritis, and diarrhea are associated symptoms. Serum calcium levels are often decreased.

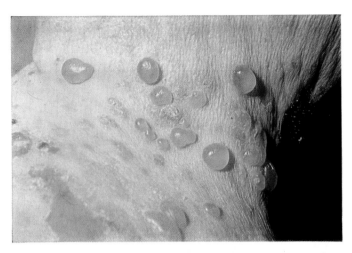

450 Pemphigus vulgaris. Large tense bullae, containing clear fluid and surrounded by clinically normal skin.

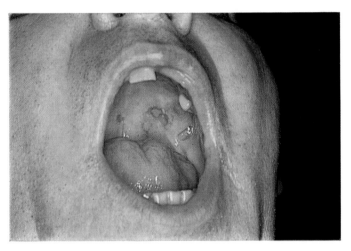

451 Pemphigus vulgaris
Bullae, mostly eroded, on the oral mucosa.

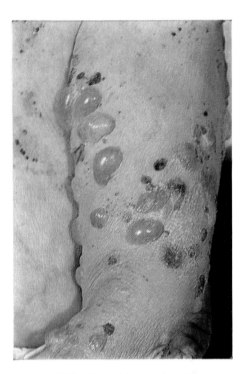

452 Pemphigus vulgaris
Clear, hemorrhagic, purulent (infected), and drying bullae arising from clinically normal skin.

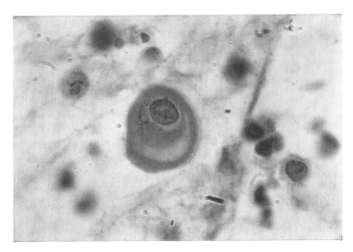

453 Pemphigus vulgaris
Typical rounded acantholytic cell with large nucleus and condensed basophilic cytoplasm.

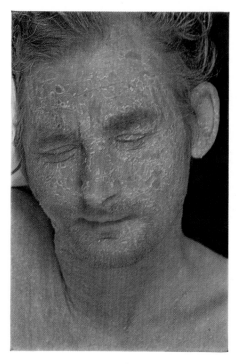

454

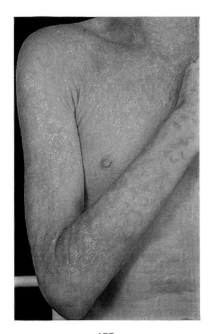

455

454 and 455   Pemphigus foliaceus
Flaking, scaly, erythematous skin without visible bullae or vesicles.

456   Pemphigus vegetans. Well circumscribed, moist, hypertrophic patches of the inguinal and genital regions. No macroscopic vesiculation.

457   Pemphigus vegetans. Fetid, purulent, vegetative masses of the genital area.

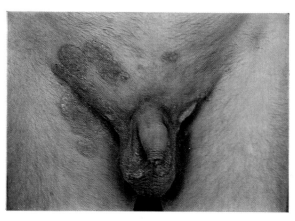

456

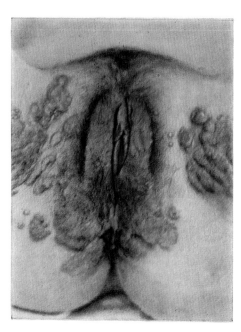

457

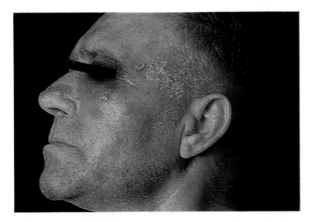

458   Pemphigus erythematosus (Senear-Usher)
Erythematous, scaling, and crusted lesions in the butterfly area of the face.

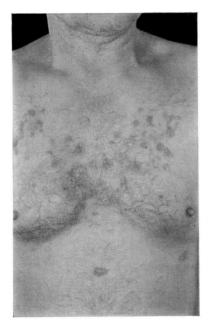

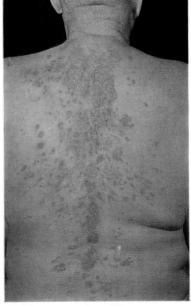

459 Pemphigus erythematosus
(Senear-Usher)
Small bullae and yellowish
crusted lesions on the chest.

460   Pemphigus erythematosus
(Senear-Usher)
Scattered, scaling, erythematous
lesions of the back.

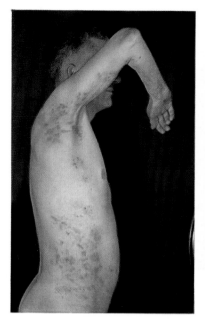

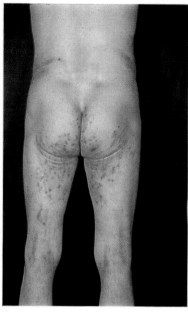

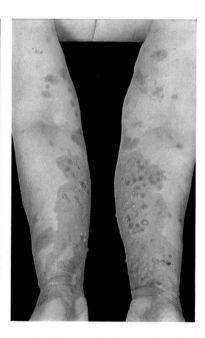

| **461** | **462** | **463 Dermatitis herpetiformis** (DUHRING) |

461 and **462 Dermatitis herpetiformis** (DUHRING)
Recurrent, symmetrical polymorphous eruption with herpetiform grouping of individual lesions in typical anatomical distribution.

463 Dermatitis herpetiformis (DUHRING)
Coalescing annular and gyrate patches, consisting of vesicles in herpetiform distribution and surrounded by inflamed erythematous skin.

464 Dermatitis herpetiformis (DUHRING)
Close-up of individual vesicular, urticarial, and erythematous lesions.

465 Dermatitis herpetiformis (DUHRING)
Pruritic gyrate wheals with central vesiculation.

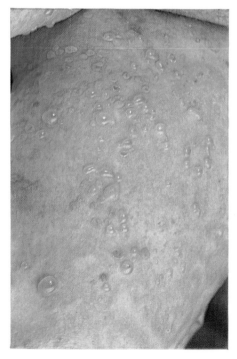

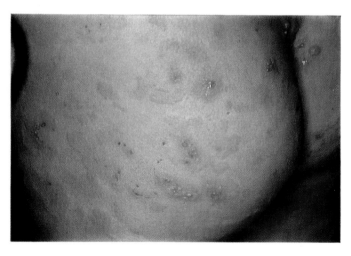

464

465

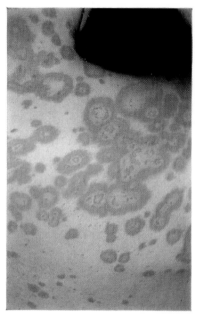

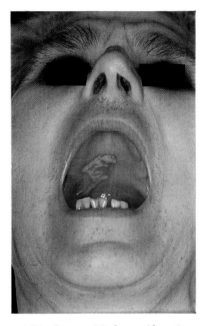

466 Dermatitis herpetiformis
(DUHRING)
Nummular, annular, and gyrate patches with new lesions in temporarily healed central zones.

467 Dermatitis herpetiformis
(DUHRING)
Eroded vesicles on the oral mucosa in herpetiform configuration.

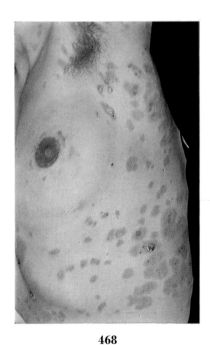

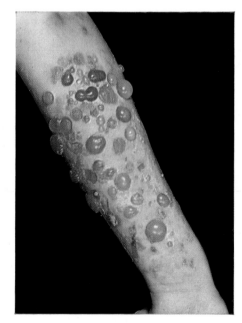

468

469

468 and 469 Herpes gestationis
Large, partially hemorrhagic blisters in a pregnant woman.

156

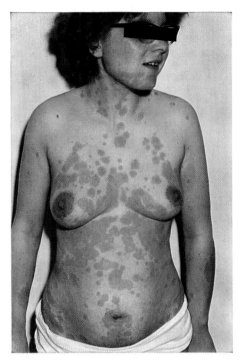

470   Herpes gestationis
Annular and gyrate, partially urticarial,
coalescing lesions and isolated vesicles.

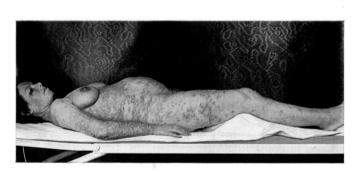

471   Impetigo herpetiformis
Widespread pustular patches in third trimester of pregnancy,
resembling pustular psoriasis.

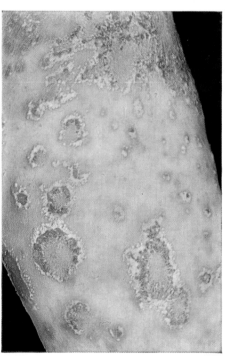

472

472   Impetigo herpetiformis. Close-up view of erythematous grouped pustules in annular arrangement.
New pustules arising predominantly in periphery of old lesions.

Vascular Reaction Patterns

Urticaria

Wheals (urticae) may be produced by toxic or allergic mechanisms. Contact with certain plants or insect bites results in localized urticarial reactions confined to the site of contact with the irritant. Urticaria distributed symmetrically over the entire integument usually is of endogenous origin (ingestants, drugs). The lesions, initially pink, turn white for a short time due to increasing osmotic pressure (compression of capillaries) in the edematous tissue, and finally become pale red wheals again. They often disappear in minutes to hours, and are followed by new lesions. Central healing or coalescence of the eruptions may produce annular or gyrate forms. Bullous or hemorrhagic wheals are seen occasionally. *Acute urticaria* is usually due to antigen-antibody reactions induced by food or drug allergens. After elimination of the causative agent, the wheals usually subside within a few days. *Chronic urticaria* is characterized by recurrent outbreaks over longer periods of time, usually without demonstrable relationship to ingestion of food or drugs.

Intestinal parasites, functional disturbances in the intestinal tract, allergens, and histamine liberators may be of etiological significance. Physical irritants, such as mechanical injury, cold, heat, and actinic effects also must be considered.

Quincke's edema (Angioneurotic edema)

Circumsribed subcutaneous edema with a sudden onset usually appears asymmetrically on normal or slightly erythematous skin. The lesions are tense but not pruritic, and have a predilection for the eyelids, lips, mucous membranes, and genitals. Drugs or foods must be considered as causative factors. In the presence of edema of the larynx, there is danger of suffocation.

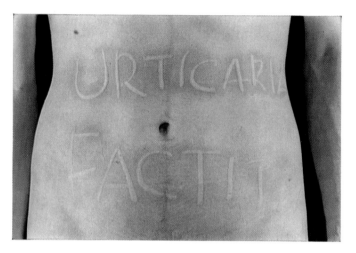

473   Factitial urticaria

Due to pressure. Raised white urticarial areas surrounded by erythematous flare.

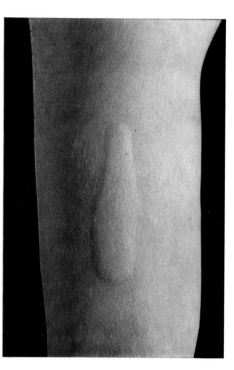

474   Cold urticaria

Induced by contact with a test tube filled with crushed ice.

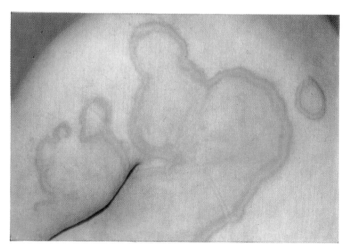

475   Acute urticaria

Annular and gyrate wheals due to penicillin hypersensitivity.

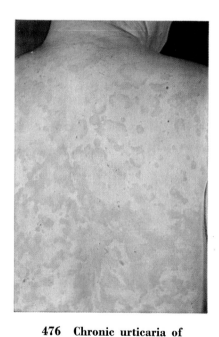

476   Chronic urticaria of unknown origin

Urticarial plaques with active borders and healing centers.

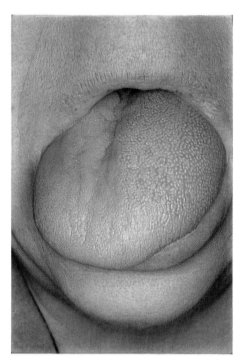

477   Quincke's edema

Massive swelling of the left portion of the tongue.

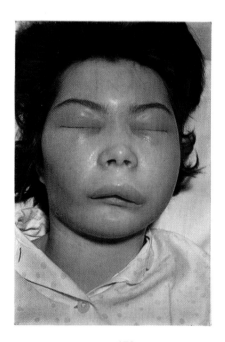

478

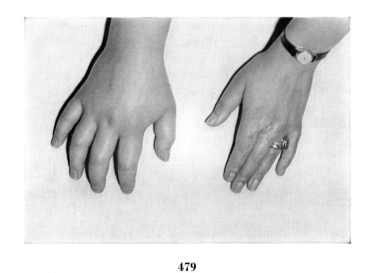

479

478 and 479   Quincke's edema

Severe circumscribed edema of the face and right hand, induced by minor mechanical trauma.
The disease had occurred in the family for four generations.

Diseases of the Cutaneous Blood Vessels

Acrocyanosis and Erythrocyanosis crurum puellarum (KLINGMÜLLER)

Both syndromes are characterized by typical persistent skin discoloration, chiefly in female patients. Endocrine disturbances are discussed as etiologic factors. In *acrocyanosis*, the clinical manifestations (bluish-pink discoloration) are arranged symmetrically and show a preference for the extensor surfaces of the hands and fingers and for the feet. The skin feels cold.

Erythrocyanosis crurum puellarum is a clinical variant of acrocyanosis. It usually involves the distal third of the lower legs of young females and is often associated with cyanosis of the acra. The discoloration ranges from pink to dark purple, making differentiation from chilblain quite difficult in some cases.

Livedo reticularis and Livedo racemosa

These are disorders of deep subcutaneous vessels.

Livedo reticularis is characterized clinically by a permanent blotchy, reticulated, livid red discoloration; etiologically, it is based on disturbances of hormonal and autonomic regulatory mechanisms. It is usually seen on the lower extremities, less often on the buttocks. The vascular changes are accentuated in cold environment.

Livedo racemosa shows an arborized pattern of bluish red discoloration. The skin alteration is due to inflammatory changes of the small arteries and veins of the subcutaneous plexus which may lead to complete occlusion. Arteriosclerosis, hypertension, periarteritis nodosa, thromboangiitis obliterans, syphilis, and tuberculosis may play a pathogenetic role in the development of livedo racemosa. Cryoglobulins may be present.

Hypertensive ischemic leg ulcers (MARTORELL)

In addition to hypertension (usually with elevated diastolic pressure), local trauma is believed to play a role in the development of this painful ulcerative disorder of middle aged females. The superficial ulcers are often surrounded by peripheral necroses. Predilection sites are the supramalleolar area and the lateral or extensor surface of the distal lower leg.

Chilblain (Pernio)

Besides the harmful effects of cold temperature (usually only a few degrees below room temperature), endogenous factors of a constitutional nature and chronic infections are operative in this disorder. Recurrent edematous, purplish, usually diffuse, nodular eruptions as well as blisters and ulcerations dominate the clinical picture. Fingers, toes, hands, feet, and lower legs are preferred areas. Cryoglobulinemia should be ruled out.

Thromboangiitis obliterans (WINIWARTER-BUERGER) (Endangiitis obliterans)

The most important symptoms of this rare inflammatory disorder of the blood vessels are intermittent claudication, diminished pulsations, discoloration, and coldness of the involved extremity. The disease starts with thickening of the intima and obliteration of the lumen by thrombi. Frequently, arterial changes are preceded by involvement of the veins in the form of *thrombophlebitis migrans*. The etiology of thromboangiitis obliterans is unknown. It has its highest incidence in men between 20 and 40 years of age, particularly in heavy smokers. Veins and arteries of the lower legs, feet, and fingers are most often affected, usually in unilateral distribution.

Allergic cutaneous vasculitis (RUITER)

Hemorrhagic or bluish red subcutaneous nodules and papulonecrotic lesions are seen in this disorder. Focal infections and drug allergies have been discussed as etiologic factors. Other forms of allergic vasculitis are *nodular dermal allergid* (Gougerot), and *erythema elevatum diutinum;* probably also *pityriasis lichenoides et varioliformis acuta* (Mucha-Habermann) and *dermatitis nodularis necrotica* (Werther-Duemling).

Arteriosclerosis obliterans
(Endangiosis arteriosclerotica)

Calcification and necrosis of the medial coat and sclerotic changes of the intima of the arteries, usually seen in men over 50 years of age, produce changes on the extremities that are difficult to differentiate clinically from thromboangiitis obliterans. In the presence of arteriosclerotic changes, diabetes mellitus should be ruled out. The most common symptoms are intermittent claudication, postural color changes, coolness, diminished pulsations, atrophy, and hair loss of the distal parts of the extremities.

Diabetic gangrene

Diabetic angiolopathy is the cause of diabetic gangrene. In most cases, only 1 or 2 toes are involved; or the gangrene may start on the dorsal aspect of the foot or on the heel. The primary lesion is a small painful nodule. Edema, exudation, and central necrosis, accompanied by a pronounced tendency to secondary infection, rapidly lead to the development of gangrenous changes. Vascular occlusion often is confined to superficial vessels.

Varicose veins and chronic venous insufficiency

Dilatation of veins in the lower extremities, especially of the medial surfaces, may be associated with or followed by *stasis dermatitis, thrombophlebitis,* sclerosis of connective tissue, pachyderma, sclerotic atrophy (*atrophie blanche* [Milian]), scarring, hyperpigmentation, petechiae, and hemosiderin deposits. The most disturbing sequelae of varicose veins are *stasis ulcers.*

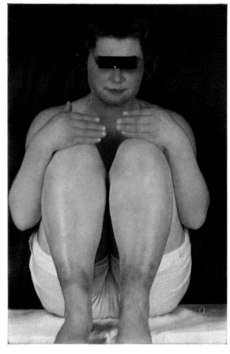

480 Erythrocyanosis crurum puellarum
Persistent brownish-violaceous discoloration of the middle and lower third of the lower legs, associated with acrocyanosis of the dorsa of the hands.

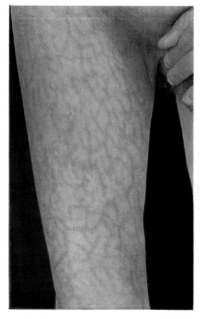

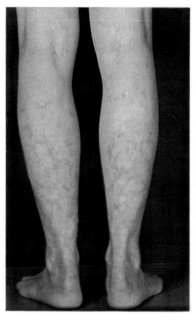

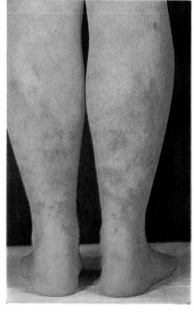

481 Livedo reticularis
Blotchy, reticulated, livid-red discoloration, accentuated by cold environment.

482 Livedo racemosa
Arborized discoloration due to arteriolar occlusion.

483 Livedo racemosa
Due to tuberculous vasculitis.

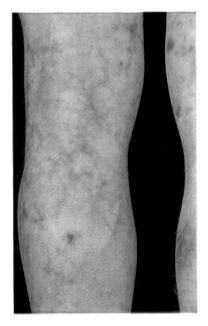

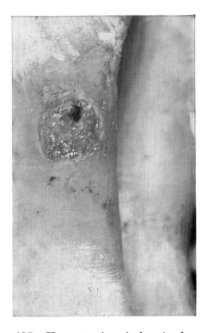

484   Livedo racemosa
Associated with periarteritis nodosa.

485   Hypertensive ischemic leg ulcer
Painful superficial ulcer in lateral supramalleolar localization, with peripheral necroses.

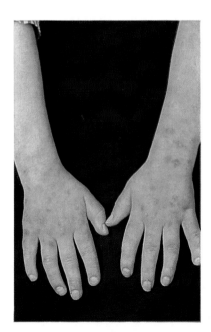

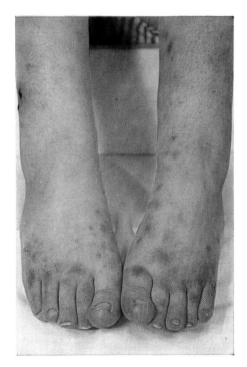

486

487

486 and 487   Chilblain (Pernio)
Diffuse purplish edematous nodules of hands and feet (in Little's syndrome).

11*

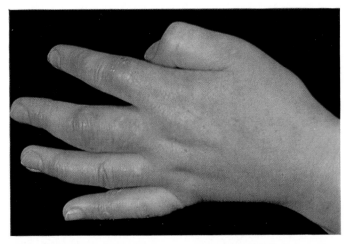

488 Chilblain (Pernio). Multiple edematous nodules of fingers.

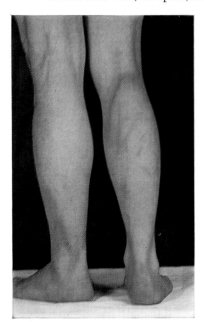

489 Thromboangiitis obliterans
Necroses in cold, atrophic, shiny skin.

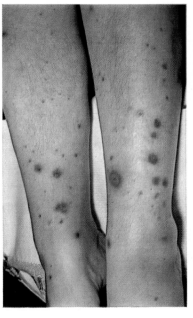

490 Thromboangiitis obliterans
Necroses of first to third finger.

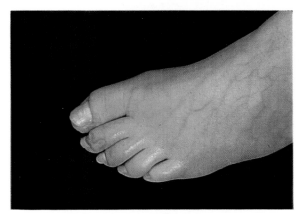

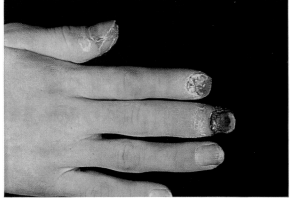

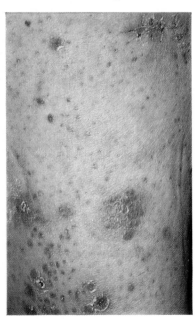

491 Phlebitis migrans
Band-like erythema
and infiltration over veins.

492 Allergic cutaneous vasculitis
Discrete red patches with necrotic
centers.

493 Nodular allergid
Crusted brownish papules and
nodules.

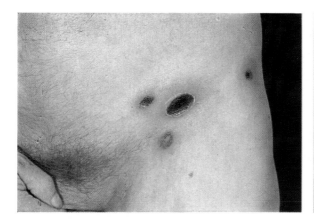

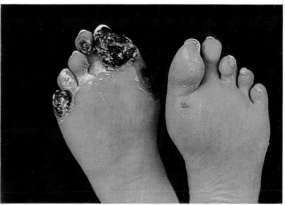

**494 Allergic cutaneous vasculitis
(dermatitis nodularis necrotica)**

Asymmetrical, tender, necrotic, inflammatory nodules. Histologic findings consistent with diagnosis.

495 Arteriosclerosis obliterans

Severe necroses of the toes, associated with diminished pulsations, coolness, and atrophy of the skin, and intermittent claudication.

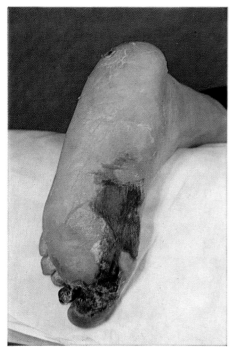

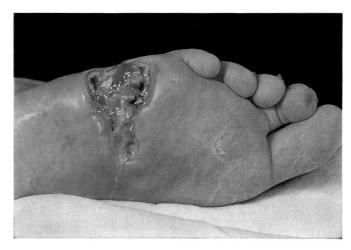

496 Diabetic gangrene
Circumscribed large necroses of the foot.

497 Diabetic gangrene
Painful, large ulcer with secondary infection.

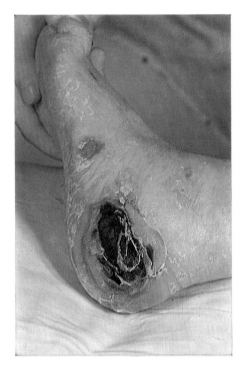

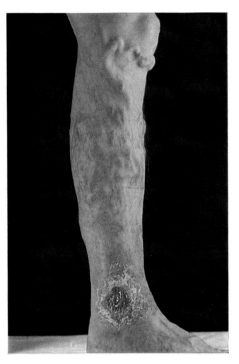

498   Diabetic gangrene
Large necrosis of heel; erythema, edema, and scaling of surrounding skin.

499   Varicose veins and stasis ulcer
Large tortuous varicose veins with recurrent stasis ulcer of medial malleolar area.

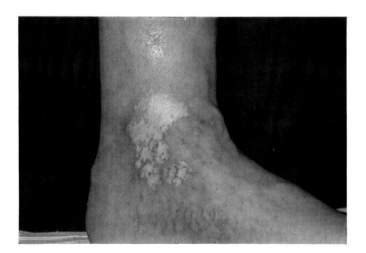

500   Atrophie blanche
Sharply circumscribed, slightly depressed, white atrophic areas associated with varicose veins.

Diseases of the Skin Appendages

Diseases of the Sebaceous Glands

Acne vulgaris

Acne usually manifests itself before and during puberty and may persist well into the third decade. The disorder affects face, chest, back, and neck, i.e., skin areas amply supplied with sebaceous glands. Increased sebum production and keratinous obstruction of the follicular orifices with comedones result in the typical clinical picture of acne which is usually polymorphous; clear-cut forms of *comedone acne, papular acne, pustular acne,* and *acne indurata* are rare. Severe forms extending deep into the cutis may heal with characteristic "ice pick" scars.

The relationship between acne vulgaris and endocrine factors is well established. Testosterone, ACTH, and cortisone and its derivatives stimulate sebum secretion and are capable of producing acne lesions in certain patients. Other etiological factors are still unknown.

In contrast to acne vulgaris, *acne conglobata* is not confined to any particular age group. It occurs predominantly in men, involving back, gluteal area, and neck, less often the face. The nuchal lesions are identical with folliculitis et perifolliculitis capitis abscedens et suffodiens. The clinical picture of acne conglobata is characterized by indolent deep-seated abscesses, ulcerations, giant or double comedones, and various types of scarring.

Acneform eruption due to drugs or occupational factors

As has been mentioned above, certain steroids are capable of inducing acne. Bromides and iodides may aggravate pre-existing acne vulgaris or induce "bromine acne" or "iodine acne," which is not preceded by comedones.

Nodular and vegetative eruptions in other areas are known as *bromoderma or iododerma tuberosum.*

Exogenous and endogenous action of chlorinated industrial products may cause severe skin changes, such as comedones, pustules, and sebum retention cysts on face, neck, chest, back, and extremities; these agents also may induce parenchymatous liver damage. Another form of occupational acne is *"oil acne"* caused by contact with mineral oils.

A peculiar form of acne is *"acne excoriée des jeunes filles"* (Brocq). The patients have a neurotic habit of picking their faces and expressing minimal acne lesions. As a result, the face is covered with numerous excoriations and flat pigmented scars. Local treatment must be supported by psychological guidance directed at normalizing the patient's behavior.

Rosacea and Rhinophyma

Rosacea is a chronic hyperemic disorder based on a seborrheic condition. It occurs chiefly in middle-aged patients. The disorder starts with vasodilation in the flush area of the face; the involved area later assumes a blotchy dusky red to purple discoloration. In addition, there are patulous follicular orifices and telangiectases on cheeks and nose, often associated with edema, greasy papules, and minute pustules. These lesions prompted the name "acne rosacea," although they are not directly related to acne vulgaris; comedones are absent. In the presence of inflammatory granulomata and marked development of papules, the disorder is called hypertrophic rosacea. Conjunctivitis and keratitis may be concomitant features. Tumorous deformation of the nose associated with marked proliferation of sebaceous glands results in the thickenes, lobulated *rhinophyma*, which is more common in men than in women.

Rosacea develops on the basis of constitutional irregularities manifested by seborrhea and disturbances of vasomotor function. It may be triggered or supported by menopause, internal diseases, achlorhydria gastric ulcers, intestinal or hepatic disorders, emotional abnormalities, ingestants (alcohol, coffee, tea, hot spices), external irritants, and local action of heat.

Differential diagnosis includes seborrheic dermatitis, acute and subacute lupus erythematosus, sarcoidosis, syphilis and tuberculosis miliaris disseminata faciei.

Granulosis rubra nasi (Jadassohn)

This rare, occasionally familial, miliaria-like disorder occurs in children and subsides during puberty. The erythematous tip of the nose is covered with beads of perspiration; papules, vesicles, pustules, and crusts are also present. The disease may be associated with persistent hyperhidrosis and diffuse redness of the face, palms, and soles.

Diseases of the Hair

Heterochromia

This may be due to an inherited circumscribed pigment anomaly of the hair, to artificial pigments, or to hair diseases such as alopecia areata, in which new hair growth may show depigmentation.

Alopecia

Congenital alopecia is irreversible; postfetal neogenesis of hair is highly unlikely. Easily confused with *alopecia congenita circumscripta* is *aplasia congenita circumscripta;* in this disorder, the skin is not developed in circumscribed areas, which have the appearance of ulcerations or scars.

Alopecia areata (Sauvage) usually has a sudden onset, occasionally preceded by headaches and neuralgia. There is complete loss of hair in sharply defined round or oval patches, usually without any visible erythema or other skin changes. In milder cases, new hair growth may occur spontaneously after 4 or 5 months. Alopecia areata usually remains confined to isolated patches of the scalp, but it may also involve the entire scalp (alopecia totalis), the beard, eyebrows, and eyelashes. In rare cases, a universal alopecia may develop. Typically, dystrophic hairs, 2 to 3 mm. long and with flattened dark tips (exclamation point hairs), surround the bald spots in alopecia areata. Dystrophic nail changes may also occur.

Telogen effluvium (Kligman) is a reversible form of hair loss. All the hairs shed (often suddenly and in great numbers) are club hairs (telogen hairs). The most common types are neonatal, postfebrile (e.g., scarlet fever), post-partum, and psychogenic effluvium. Some drugs, especially heparinoids, may also induce telogen effluvium. Hair loss usually starts 6 to 12 weeks following the onset of the stress situation. Regrowth may not occur for several months. (Normal hair of the scalp grows 3 mm. in 10 days.)

Dystrophic anagen effluvium is another type of reversible hair loss with predominantly dystrophic anagen hairs. It is seen as a side effect of chemotherapy with cytotoxic drugs, or after systemic poisons. Hair loss usually starts shortly after the injury; it is often more massive than telogen effluvium and may involve almost all growing hair follicles.

Cicatricial alopecia is an irreversible process due to destruction of the hair papillae by local trauma or by chronic inflammatory or scarring diseases of the scalp, (e.g., chronic radiodermatitis, scleroderma, chronic discoid lupus erythematosus, lupus vulgaris, lichen planus, folliculitis decalvans, and follicular infections).

Pseudopelade (Brocq) is characterized by marked atrophy of the scalp and loss of hair follicles in multiple coin-sized irregular patches with finger-like projections and "onion skin" surface. Some authors believe pseudopelade to be identical with follicular atrophic lichen planus (lichen planopilaris) of the scalp (Graham-Little syndrome).

Disorders of the Nails

Pits, furrows, streaks, or bands of the nail plate may be caused by external or internal factors. The actual time of the injury can be estimated as follows: the normal nail grows 1 mm. in 10 days. Eight weeks pass until the new nail becomes visible; 5 to 6 months until the distal end is reached. It should be considered, however, that the rate of nail growth varies in different periods of life, and that fingernails always grow faster than toenails.

Pitted nails

Tiny surface pits of the nail plate are characteristic of psoriasis, but also may be associated with dermatitis, alopecia areata, and other disorders involving the nail matrix.

Nail changes in psoriasis arthropathica

Deformities of hands and feet are usually associated with severe dystrophic changes of the nail plate.

169

Clubbing of the nails (Hippocratic nails)

Clubbed fingers and the associated clubbing, thickening, and increased convexity of the nails are seen primarily in chronic pulmonary and cardiac disorders.

Transverse furrows (Beau's lines)

Severe systemic stress (febrile infectious diseases, allergic or toxic disorders, nutritional deficiencies, severe shock, and local trauma or skin diseases) may cause temporary impairment of nail growth manifested in shallow or deep transverse furrows or grooves.

Mees' lines

Mees' lines are a variety of leukonychia striata in which a single white transverse band can be observed in all the nails. It used to be seen following arsenic or thallium poisoning, but it may also occur in febrile illnesses, Hodgkin's disease, severe cardiac disorders and many other systemic diseases.

Leukonychia

Total or partial chalky white discoloration of the smooth, sometimes unusually soft nail plate may occur following incorrect manicuring.

Spoon nails (Koilonychia; Ball-Heller)

Thin concave nails with rough distal edges may be associated with achlorhydric anemia and concomitant gastrointestinal disorders. Familial incidence and traumatic origin of koilonychia have been reported.

Longitudinal ridges

Accentuation of the normal longitudinal ridges of the nail plate is primarily a senile manifestation. Longitudinal fractures or splitting of the nail plate occur less frequently and are independent of age. Chronic radiodermatitis may induce similar nail changes. Occupational factors are also important.

Onycholysis

Gradual separation of the nail plate from the nail bed starting at the distal edge results in a halfmoon or pocket shaped free space beneath the whitish nail plate. This may be due to various external factors, such as moist work, alkalis, and faulty manicuring techniques.

Subungual hyperkeratoses

Subungual hyperkeratoses with separation of the nail plate may be associated with chronic dermatitis, psoriasis, pityriasis rubra pilaris, onychomycosis, and occasionally, with allergic reactions to local anesthetics used by dentists and ophthalmologists.

Onychogryphosis

Claw-like deformation of the nails, usually limited to the large toe nails, is not infrequently seen in older patients. The nails are hard and markedly thickened, twisted and curved. Simultaneously, there is marked subungual hyperkeratosis. Local pressure, deformities of the foot, and local circulatory disturbances may be responsible for this abnormality. Claw nails on the fingers are rare.

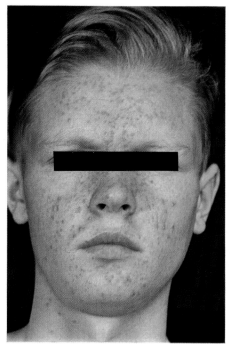

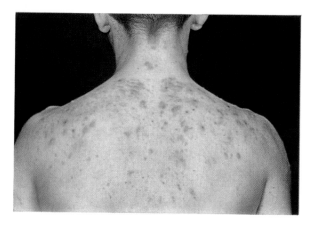

501 Acne vulgaris

Many papules, with some pustules and comedones in characteristic localization.

502 Acne vulgaris

Infiltrated papules and nodules with some scarring of the upper back.

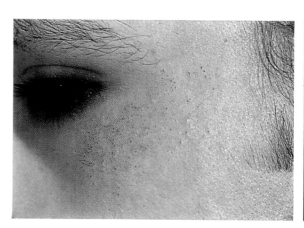

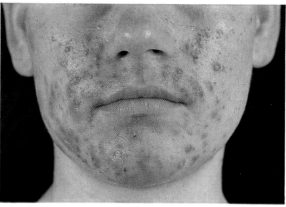

503 Acne vulgaris (comedone acne)

Numerous dark follicular comedones; no inflammatory lesions.

504 Acne vulgaris (acne indurata)

Deeply indurated, nodular, papular, and pustular lesions with characteristic small "ice pick" scars.

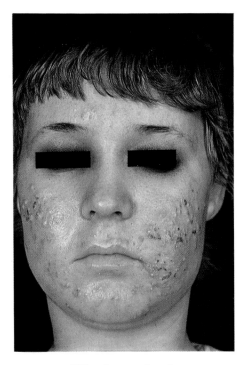

505   Acne vulgaris
Numerous superficial and deep erythematous pustules and indurated
inflamed cystic lesions of the chin and cheeks.

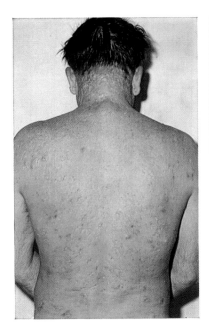

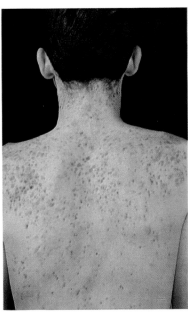

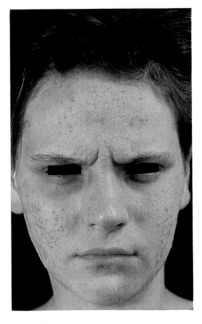

506   Acne conglobata
Deep-seated indolent abscesses
resulting in severe scarring. Often
associated with large comedones.

507   Steroid acne
Severe acne with large papules
and comedones induced by
corticosteroid therapy.

508   Occupational acne
In worker exposed to fumes of
chloronaphthalene.

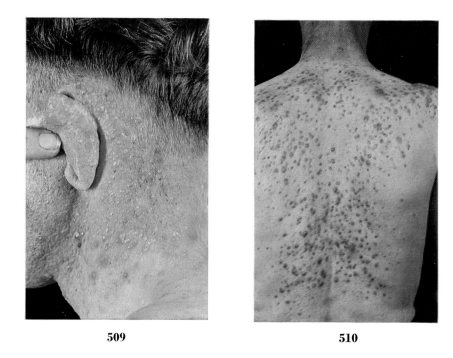

509   510

509 and **510**   **Occupational acne**

Severe eruption with numerous comedones, papules, pustules and retention
cysts due to exposure to tetrachlordibenzodioxin.

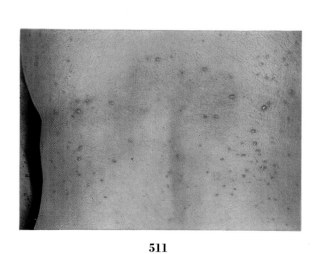

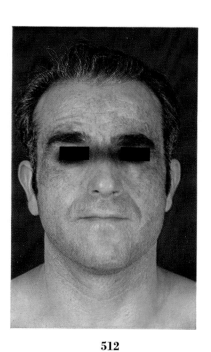

511   512

511 and **512**   **Oil acne**

Face, trunk, and extremities show typical changes induced by oil-soaked work clothes.
Obstruction of the follicular orifices by dark comedones and dirt particles; secondary pustule
formation.

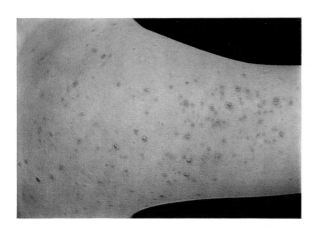

513 Bromide acne

Crusted papulopustular eruption of the shoulders.

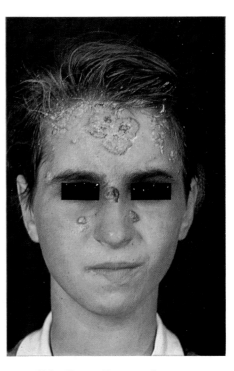

514 Bromoderma tuberosum

Circumscribed nodular and vegetative crusted lesions of the face.

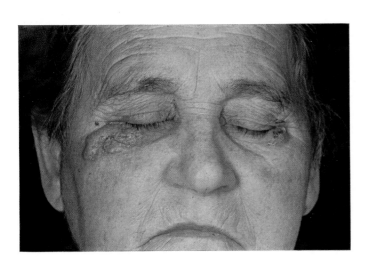

515

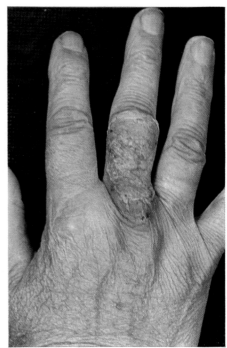

516

515 and 516 Iododerma tuberosum

Large, raised, erythematous, crusted vegetations with verrucous surface under both eyes and on the dorsum of the finger.

174

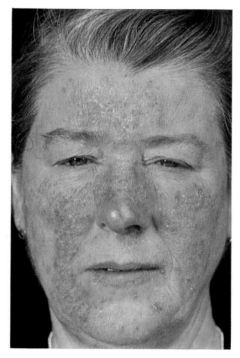

517 Rosacea

Erythema, papular infiltration, slight
desquamation, blepharitis, and conjunctivitis. No comedones.

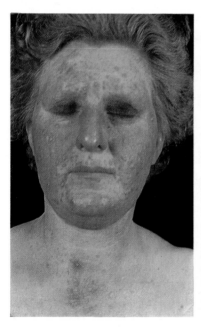

518 Rosacea

Severe pustular eruption. Marked
erythema and infiltration; numerous small pustules. No comedones.

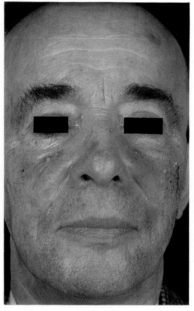

519 Lupoid rosacea

Infiltrated lesions of the cheeks.
No histologic evidence of cutaneous tuberculosis.

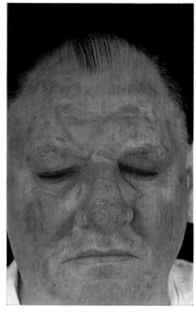

520 Rosacea

With hypertrophic changes of the
forehead, cheeks, and nose.

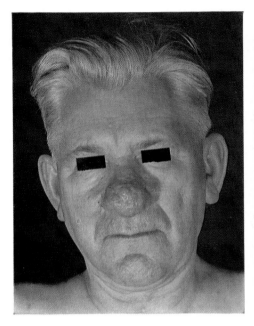

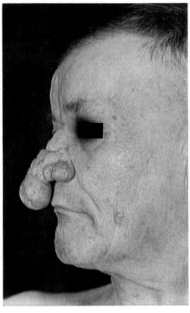

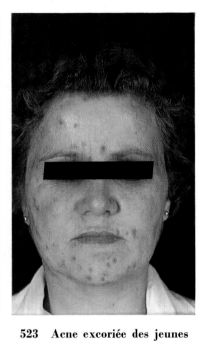

521 Rhinophyma

Lobulated proliferation of the nose in a patient with rosacea.

522 Rhinophyma

Grotesque, lobulated, proliferative growth of the nose in a patient with rosacea.

523 Acne excoriée des jeunes filles

Multiple excoriations and small scars due to neurotic habit of picking minimal acne lesions.

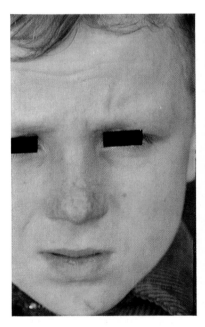

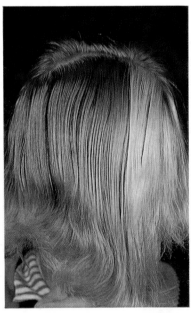

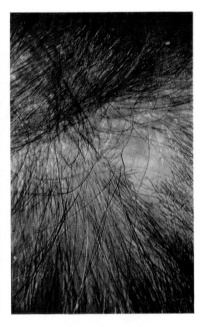

524 Granulosis rubra nasi

Erythema and small vesicles on the tip of the nose.

525 Heterochromia of scalp hair

On the right, a large almost white strand of hair; on the left, a narrow black one.

526 Congenital circumscribed aplasia of the scalp

With permanent alopecia and scarring.

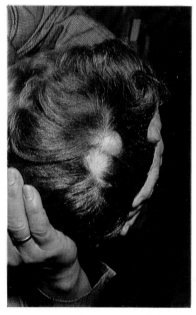

527   Alopecia areata
Round patch of alopecia areata adjacent to circumscribed alopecia caused by a sebaceous cyst.

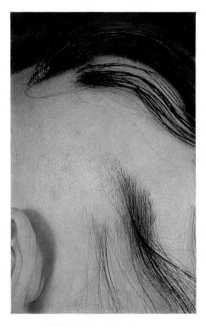

528   Alopecia areata
No atrophy; the follicular orifices are clearly visible. Some short "exclamation point" hairs in center of the picture.

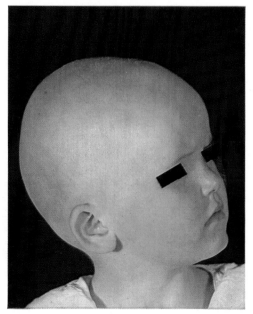

529   Alopecia areata
Total alopecia with loss of scalp hairs, eyebrows and eyelashes.

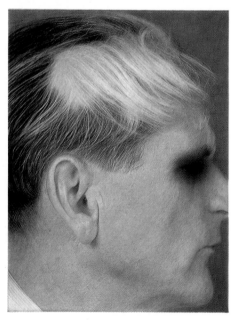

530   Alopecia areata
Regrowth of nonpigmented hairs.

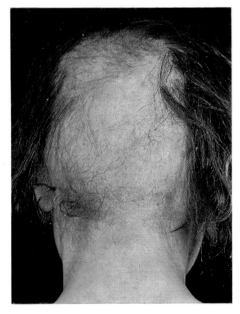

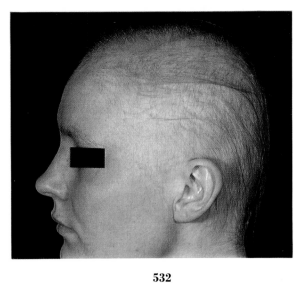

531   **532**

531 and 532   Anagen effluvium

Almost complete hair loss following ingestion of rat poison containing thallium.
Most hairs show dystrophic anagen hair roots. In contrast to telogen effluvium, hair loss starts
shortly after injury.

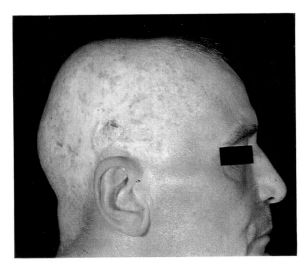

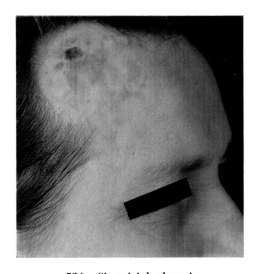

533   Cicatricial alopecia

Associated with chronic radiodermatitis following
x-ray treatment of "cradle cap" 52 years earlier.

534   Cicatricial alopecia

Associated with radiation ulcer following x-ray treatment of lupus vulgaris.

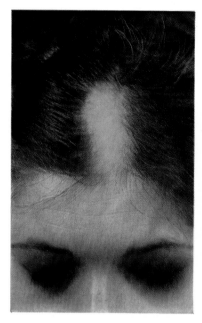

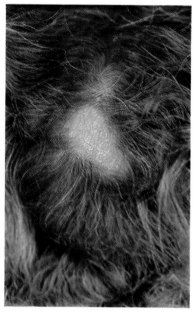

535 Cicatricial alopecia

Circumscribed scleroderma
of scalp and forehead
("en coup de sabre").

536 Cicatricial alopecia

Chronic discoid lupus erythematosus with circumscribed alopecia, erythema, scaling, follicular plugs, and atrophy.

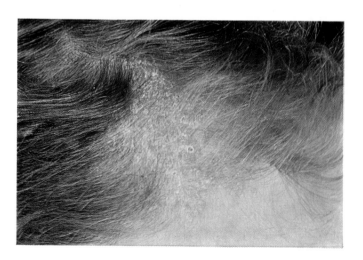

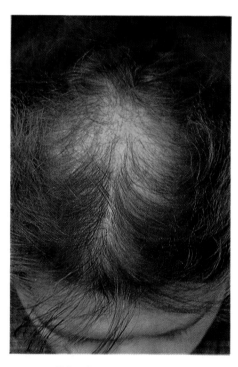

537 Cicatricial alopecia

Lupus vulgaris with erythema, infiltration, scaling, and
partial alopecia.

538 Cicatricial alopecia

Atrophic lichen planus of the scalp
(GRAHAM-LITTLE syndrome).

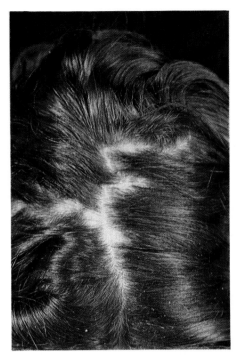

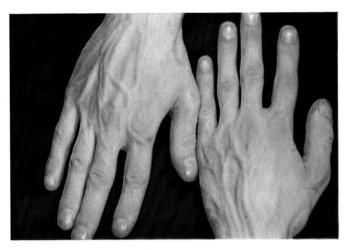

539   Pseudopelade (Brocq)

Multiple, irregular, atrophic patches with finger-like projections and "onion-skin" surface.

540   Clubbing of the nails (hippocratic nails)

Thickening and increased convexity of the nails.

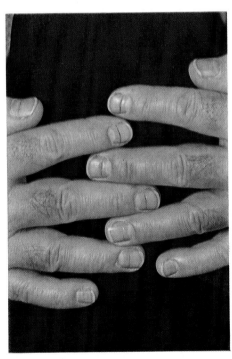

541   Transverse furrows (Beau's lines)

Shallow transverse grooves of the nails following febrile infectious disease.

180

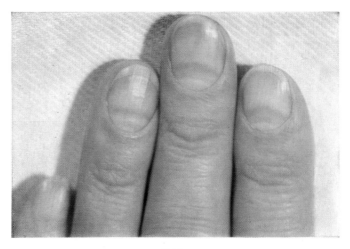

542

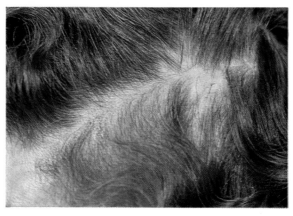

543

542 and **543** **Transverse furrows (Beau's lines)**
The nail changes followed heparin treatment and were accompanied by massive diffuse loss
of telogen hairs (telogen effluvium).

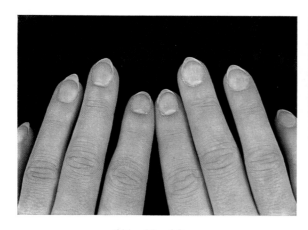

544 Mees' lines
Lunula-colored, whitish, transverse bands due
to thallium poisoning.

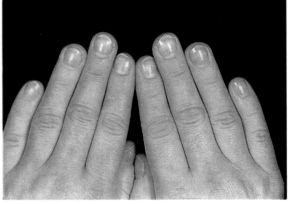

545 Mees' lines
Whitish bands due to thallium poisoning.

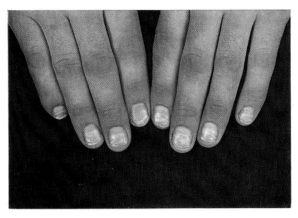

546   Partial leukonychia
Spotty whitish discoloration of the nails.

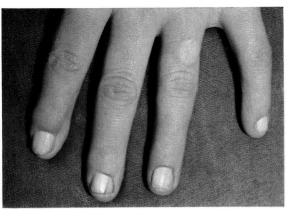

547   Total leukonychia
Chalky discoloration of all the fingernails.

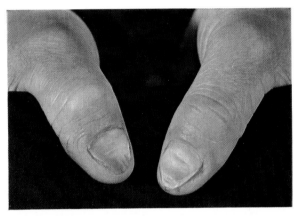

548   Spoon nails (koilonychia). Thin concave nails with rough distal edges.

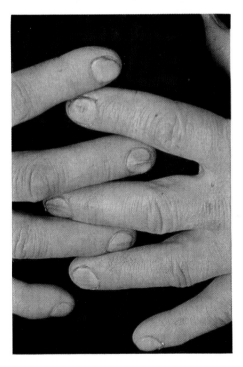

549   Longitudinal ridges of the fingernails

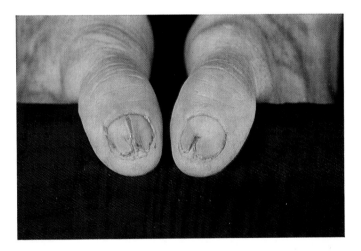

550   Longitudinal ridges
With fissures of the nail plate, exposing the nail bed in some areas (same patient as shown in fig. 549).

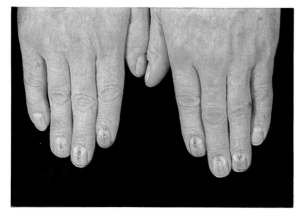

551   Medial canaliform dystrophy of the fingernails

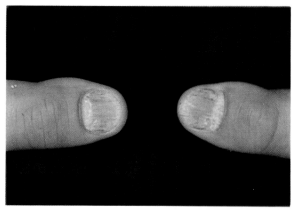

552   Onychorrhexis
Breakage and longitudinal splitting of the nails.

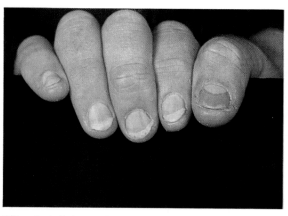

553   Onycholysis. Distal whitish discoloration due to separation of the nail plate from the nail bed.

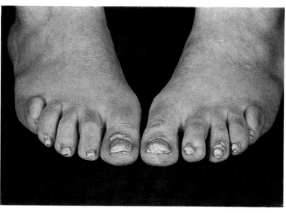

554   Psoriatic nails
Whitish dislocation, brittleness, and subungual hyperkeratotic debris.

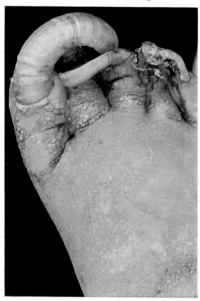

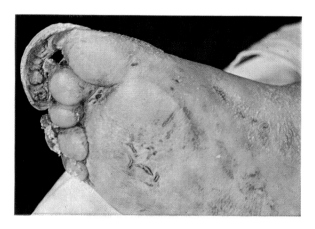

555

556

555 and **556   Onychogryphosis.** Thickening and claw-like deformation of toenails.

Diseases of the Corium

(Atrophic and hypertrophic changes of the dermis)

Chronic actinic skin changes
(Farmer's skin; cutis rhomboidalis nuchae)

Persons habitually exposed to sunlight and other climatic influences may develop premature senile degenerative changes of the skin. Atrophy, dryness, loss of elasticity, wrinkling, pigmentary changes, telangiectases, circumscribed hyperkeratoses, and precancerous skin changes belong to the symptomatology of this disorder. *Cutis rhomboidalis nuchae* is a special form of farmer's skin. This abnormality, which occurs predominantly in men, is characterized by thickening and hyperpigmentation of the skin and exaggeration of the normal skin markings on the back of the neck. Persistent exposure to the sun is the main cause of this alteration.

Striae atrophicae (Striae distensae)

Slightly depressed, bluish-red (later white), shiny smooth atrophic lines in a parallel or fan-shaped arrangement may occur in the abdominal region, on the buttocks, the thighs, and the breasts in association with pregnancy or rapid growth, during or following weight reduction in obesity, in some systemic infections, after long-term corticosteroid treatment, and in Cushing's syndrome. In all these instances, the striae are attributed to increased cortisone production of the adrenal cortex; stretching is believed to play only a secondary role.

Atrophoderma reticulata (Darier)
(Atrophoderma vermiculata)

In prepubertal patients, both cheeks may show flat, polygonal depressed, atrophic pit-like lesions in a symmetrical, reticulated arrangement. These lesions give the skin a worm-eaten appearance.

Anetoderma (Macular atrophy)

This is a circumscribed, sharply defined, round or oval form of macular atrophy with oft bag-like protrusions. Lesions beginning with inflammatory macules are referred to as the *erythematous type* (Jadassohn); initially urticarial reactions are characteristic of the Pellizzari *type*. Hernia-like protrusions of flaccid skin without visible preceding inflammation are known as the Schwenninger-Buzzi *type*. Secondary anetoderma may follow various systemic diseases, e.g., syphilis, measles, lupus erythematosus and sarcoidosis.

Acrodermatitis chronica atrophicans
(Pick-Herxheimer)
(Diffuse idiopathic atrophy)

This disease is seen predominantly on the dorsa of hands and feet, as well as on the forearms and lower legs of women over 40 years of age. An initial inflammatory-edematous stage is followed by an atrophic stage. The skin is easily movable and resembles crumpled cigarette paper; it becomes transparent due to loss of subcutaneous fatty tissue. Deeper blood vessels and tendons become visible, and telangiectases contribute to the characteristic clinical picture of the disease. Late changes include deep fibroid nodules (juxta-articular nodules) and sclerotic areas, often in the form of linear fibrotic bands, predominantly on the lower legs and in the ulnar region. Secondary ulceration, regional lymphadenopathy, dysproteinemia, and increased sedimentation rate complete the symptomatology of Herxheimer's disease. Its cause is unknown.

Poikiloderma vasculare atrophicans (Jacobi)

This very rare, slowly progressive syndrome may occur as a secondary poikiloderma associated with other diseases (dermatomyositis, scleroderma), or occur independently as *primary congenital poikiloderma*. Symmetric atrophy, telangiectases, and mottled hyperpigmentation are the most prominent symptoms, often simulating chronic radiodermatitis. In some cases it has preceded leukemias and lymphomas. It may affect any region of the skin.

Lichen sclerosus et atrophicus

This disorder may simulate guttate scleroderma or atrophic lichen planus. Its histological and clinical characteristics, however, warrant its classification as a disease entity that may be identical with white spot disease.

Thin, wrinkled, ivory-white, atrophic and sclerotic macules and grouped, polygonal, flat-topped white papules with central delling and follicular plugging may be disseminated over the entire body surface, but usually are confined to the upper trunk and neck or the genital area. In female patients, this leads to the clinical picture of *kraurosis vulvae*, a chronic sclerotic pruritic process of the vulva, with parchment-like whitish skin changes. In men a similar condition is called *kraurosis penis* or *balanitis xerotica obliterans*. The atrophic process involves the glans and the prepuce. It may obstruct the urinary stream and require surgical treatment.

Localized scleroderma (Morphea)

Morphea is most common on the trunk of young patients and takes a benign course. The disease starts with a round or oval, circumscribed, slightly erythematous, smooth plaque with a firm white sclerotic center. The lesion spreads peripherally and is surrounded by a typical violaceous halo. The skin appendages in the involved areas become atrophic.

Linear forms are seen on forehead and scalp (en coup de sabre) and on the extremities; they may be associated with atrophy of muscle and bone.

Diffuse systemic sclerosis
(Progressive systemic scleroderma)

Progressive or *diffuse systemic scleroderma* has a grave prognosis. Involving the connective tissue and the blood vessels, the disease manifests itself not only on the skin, but also in internal organs (esophagus, lungs, heart, kidney, skeletal system).

From the dermatological aspect, the clinical picture is dominated by typical sclerodermic changes, associated with hyperpigmentation, atrophic ulcers, and telangiectases, particularly on the hands (claw-like fingers), feet, and neck. The face is expressionless due to restricted mobility.

Dermatomyositis (Wagner-Unverricht)

This grave disease is more common in middle aged females; it involves skin and muscles, especially of the face, neck, arms, and legs. Nonspecific diffuse or macular, often edematous, mostly symmetrically arranged erythematous lesions usually appear first on the face — frequently with characteristic "heliotrope bloating" of the upper eyelids. Weakness, tenderness, and atrophy of shoulder and hip muscles are suggestive symptoms. The disease may take a rapidly progressive or a chronic course (often with calcinosis cutis); spontaneous cures with atrophy or induration have been observed. In most cases there is involvement of internal organs (heart, lungs, intestinal tract, kidneys). The most common fatal complication is interstitial pneumonitis or bronchopneumonia. Internal neoplasms (usually adenocarcinomas) should be ruled out in all adult patients with dermatomyositis.

The poikilodermatic type runs a more chronic course. Pigmentary changes, diffuse atrophy, and telangiectasia are its characteristics. The high mortality rate of dermatomyositis apparently can be reduced somewhat by the use of corticosteroids and antibiotics.

Chronic discoid lupus erythematosus

In chronic discoid lupus erythematosus, sharply outlined inflammatory, nonpruritic, erythematous, scaling plaques with follicular hyperkeratoses spread peripherally, leaving central atrophy, telangiectasia and scarring. The disease is aggravated by sunlight, and is usually seen in exposed areas of the face (often in characteristic "butterfly" distribution), ears, neck, scalp, and arms. Its incidence is highest in middle aged persons, somewhat higher in women than in men. In rare cases, multiple typical discoid patches may occur on the trunk and other body areas in the form of a widespread, disseminate, chronic discoid lupus erythematosus. The etiology of the disease is unknown; systemic symptoms are usually absent.

Acute systemic lupus erythematosus
(Kaposi-Libman-Sacks syndrome)

Very rarely, acute systemic lupus erythematosus may evolve from chronic discoid lupus erythematosus; usually, it occurs without preceding skin changes. The disease involves connective tissue and vasculature, and has a higher incidence in young females than in males. It starts with erythematous patches on the face and the hands (fingertips), accompanied by fever and malaise. The symptomatology of acute systemic lupus erythematosus also includes endocarditis, polyserositis myalgia, arthritis, glomerulonephritis, central nervous system disorders (convulsions), and mucous membrane involvement. Hematologic findings include leukopenia, lupus erythematosus (L. E.) cells (HARGRAVES) and the L. E. factor (HASERICK). The disease usually takes an intermittent clinical course. Remissions may be obtained with corticosteroids and antibiotics. In general, the prognosis is unfavorable, although subacute and chronic cases extending over 10 to 20 years have been reported. Autoimmunization reactions are believed to play a role in the pathogenesis of the disease.

Lipodystrophy

Lipodystrophy, presenting as an atrophic depressed skin area due to loss of subcutaneous fat, may develop from a lipophagic granuloma induced by local trauma (mechanical injury, injection). Insulin lipodystrophy is the best known form of this disorder.

Subcutaneous fat necrosis of the newborn (CAUSE)
(Adiponecrosis subcutanea neonatorum)

In otherwise healthy newborn babies, livid skin discoloration may appear several days or weeks after birth, with sharply circumscribed areas of rubbery hardening in the subcutaneous fatty tissue. The disorder is often self-limited. It usually resolves spontaneously through softening and absorption or discharge of amorphous fatty masses. This abnormality of the fatty tissue is frequently due to pressure or to cold.

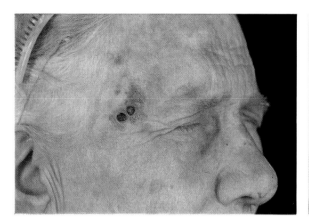

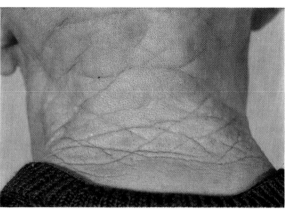

557   Chronic actinic skin changes (Farmer's skin)
Atrophy, wrinkling, dryness, and pigmentary and hyperkeratotic changes complicated by a senile keratosis with malignant degeneration on the temple.

558   Cutis rhomboidalis nuchae
Thickening and hyperpigmentation of nuchal skin with exaggeration of normal surface markings.

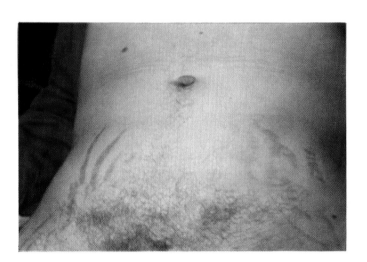

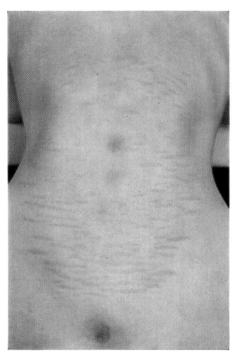

559   Striae atrophicae
In an obese male with diabetes mellitus.

560   Striae atrophicae
Bluish-red, slightly depressed, smooth atrophic lines on the abdomen in parallel arrangement.

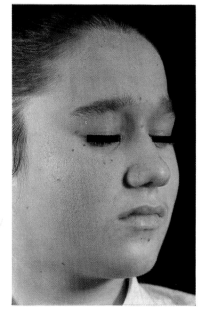

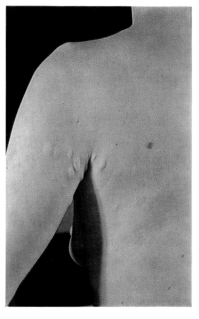

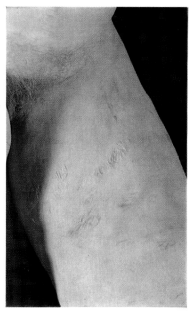

561 Atrophoderma reticulata

Small, pit-like, polygonal, atrophic depressions of the cheek in reticulated arrangement.

562 Anetoderma
(SCHWENNINGER-BUZZI)

Sharply defined, soft, oval, hernia-like protrusions of flaccid skin. No visible preceding inflammation.

563 Anetoderma
(JADASSOHN)

Sharply defined, wrinkled atrophic areas with "crumpled cigarette paper" surface. Preceded by erythematous macules.

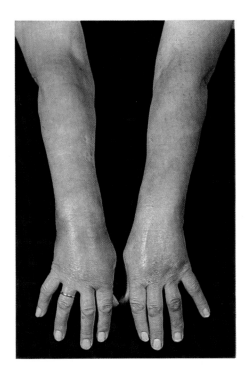

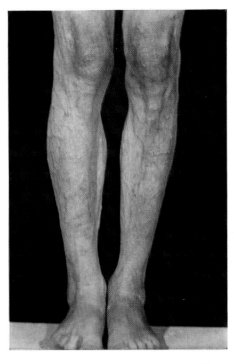

564 Acrodermatitis chronica atrophicans
(PICK-HERXHEIMER). Early, inflammatory, edematous stage with beginning "cigarette paper" atrophy of the dorsa of the hands.

565 Acrodermatitis chronica atrophicans
(PICK-HERXHEIMER). Advanced atrophic stage. Veins are clearly visible through transparent skin.

188

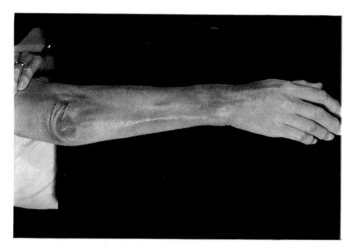

566   Acrodermatitis chronica atrophicans (Pick-Herxheimer)
Band-like, inflammatory infiltration (ulnar band).

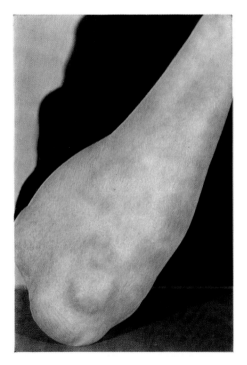

**567   Acrodermatitis chronica atrophi-
cans** (Pick-Herxheimer)
With fibrotic juxta-articular node.

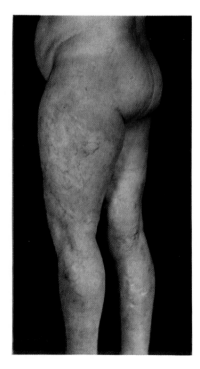

**568   Acrodermatitis chronica atrophi-
cans** (Pick-Herxheimer)
Deep vessels are clearly visible.

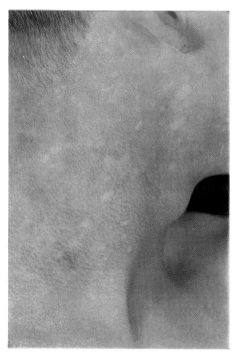

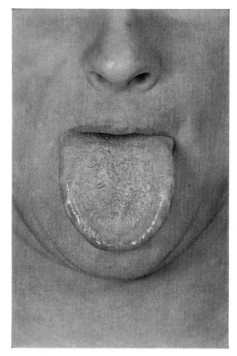

569

570

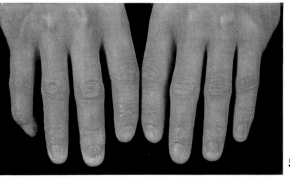

571

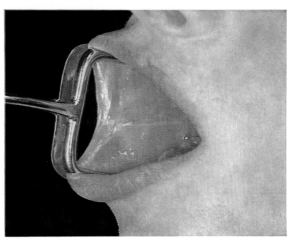

572

569, 570, 571 and **572   Poikiloderma vasculare atrophicans** (Jacobi)

A case of "primary congenital poikiloderma." In addition to skin changes (depigmented atrophic lesions, reticulated pigmentation, lichenoid papules, telangiectases), leukoplakia of the tongue, telangiectasia of the oral mucosa, and onychorrhexis of the nails were present.

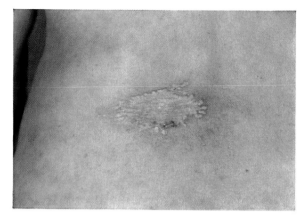

573   Lichen sclerosus et atrophicus

Grouped, flat-topped, polygonal, ivory-white, atrophic
papules with central delling on lower back.

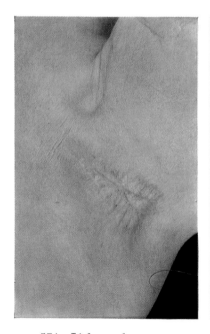

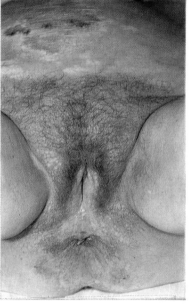

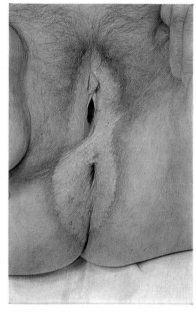

**574   Lichen sclerosus et
atrophicus**

Confluent, thick, wrinkled, atrophic and sclerotic macular lesions
of the neck.

**575   Lichen sclerosus et
atrophicus**

Extensive involvement of the abdomen, vulva, and anal region.

**576   Lichen sclerosus et
atrophicus**

Involvement of genital region
(kraurosis vulvae) and anus.

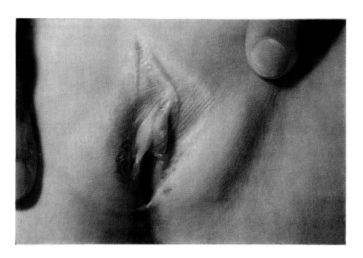

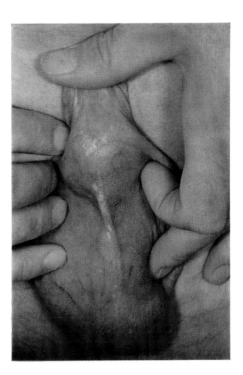

577 Lichen sclerosus et atrophicus
Parchment-like, whitish, sclerotic changes of the vulva in
an infant.

578 Lichen sclerosus et atrophicus
Discrete and patchy white atrophic
areas of male genitals.

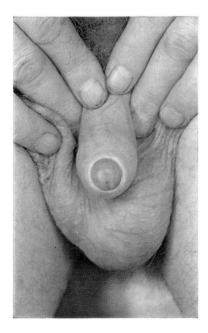

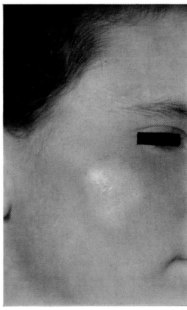

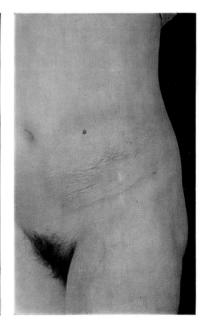

**579 Lichen sclerosus et
atrophicus**
Atrophy of prepuce and glans
penis (kraurosis penis; balanitis
xerotica obliterans).

580 Localized scleroderma
Circumscribed smooth plaque
with firm white sclerotic center
surrounded by erythematous violaceous halo (morphea).

581 Localized scleroderma
Large, firm, whitish plaques with
violaceous halo on lower abdomen.

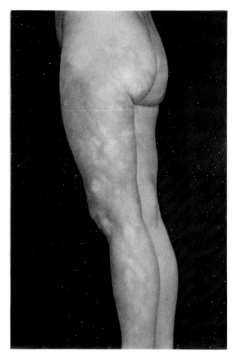

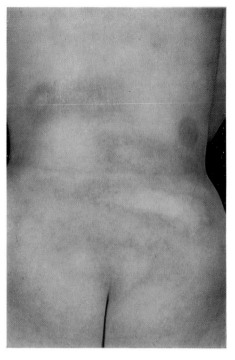

582   Localized scleroderma

Numerous firm white areas surrounded
by erythematous purplish skin extending over the entire left leg.

583   Localized scleroderma

Older plaques show peripheral hyperpigmentation; active lesions are characterized by violaceous border.

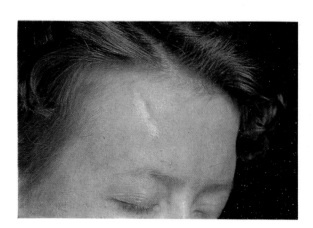

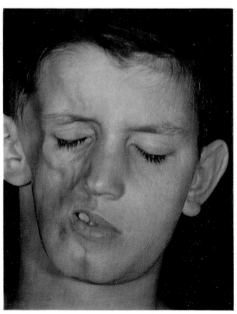

584   Localized scleroderma (en coup de sabre)

Linear lesion on forehead resembling saber scar.

585   Facial hemiatrophy

With localized scleroderma and involvement of the osseous system.

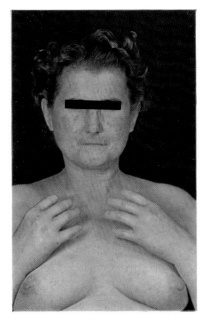

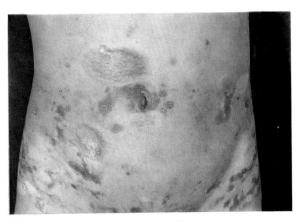

586   Diffuse systemic sclerosis
Restricted mobility of the face, numerous telangiectases, claw-like fingers (sclerodactylia).

587   Localized scleroderma, lichen planus, lichen sclerosus et atrophicus, and vitiligo
Occurring simultaneously in a patient with active pulmonary tuberculosis.

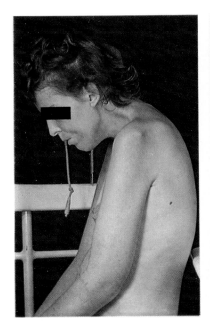

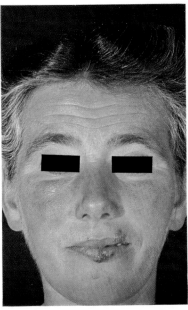

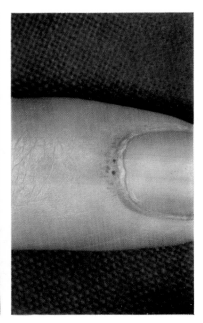

588   Dermatomyositis
Characteristic posture and facial expression of a patient suffering from severe dermatomyositis.

589   Dermatomyositis
Butterfly-shaped heliotrope discoloration of the face.

590   Dermatomyositis
Vascular ectasias, punctate atrophy, and hemorrhagic necroses of the nail fold (HEUCK-GOTTRON sign).

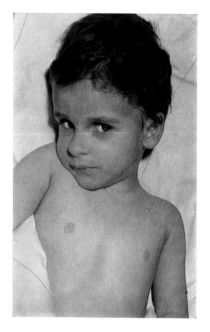

591

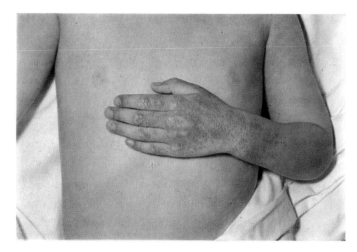

592

591 and 592   Dermatomyositis
Marked edema of the upper lip, diffuse erythema of the face, macular erythema of the shoulders, arms, and upper chest. On the dorsal aspects of the hands, circumscribed atrophic patches, telangiectases, pigmentary changes, and lichenoid papules (poikilodermic type).

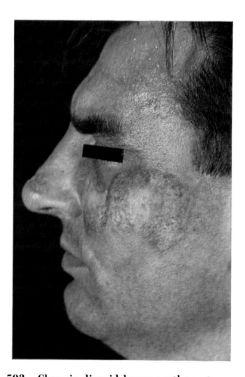

593   Chronic discoid lupus erythematosus
Sharply outlined, erythematous, scaling plaque with central atrophy,
follicular hyperkeratoses, telangiectases, and pigmentary changes in the "butterfly area" of the face.

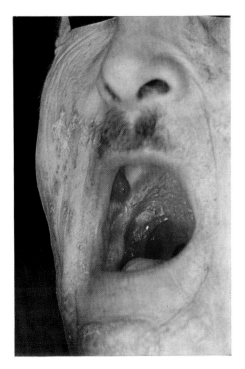

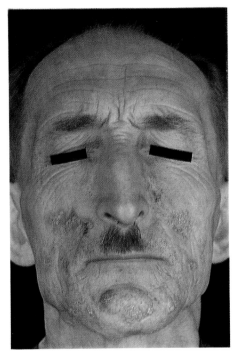

594   **595**

594 and 595   Chronic discoid lupus erythematosus

Hyperkeratotic lesions of the face and erythematous patches with reticulated, grayish-white discoloration of the oral mucosa.

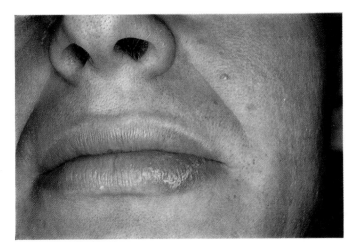

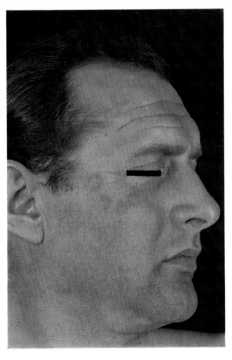

596   Chronic discoid lupus erythematosus

Atrophy and whitish discoloration of the lower lip.

597   Chronic discoid lupus erythematosus

Early, sharply defined, disk-shaped, erythematous, hypersensitive infiltrations with atrophic centers.

13*

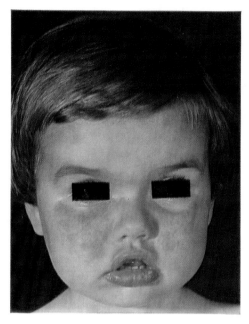

598 Chronic discoid lupus erythematosus

Butterfly-shaped erythema of the cheeks and involvement
of the lips in a child.

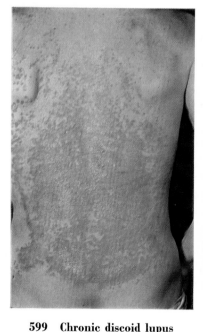

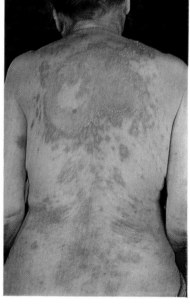

**599 Chronic discoid lupus
erythematosus**

Disseminated form, with discrete
and confluent erythematous scaling patches.

**600 Subacute lupus
erythematosus**

Acute exacerbation of chronic
discoid lupus erythematosus involving large areas of the back.

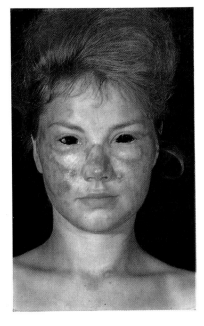

601 Subacute lupus erythematosus
In stage of acute exacerbation with marked erythematous patches of the face.

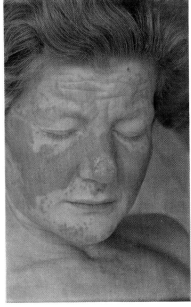

602 Acute systemic lupus erythematosus
Erythematous patches of the butterfly area of the face accompanied by fever and systemic symptoms.

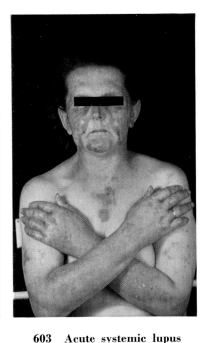

603 Acute systemic lupus erythematosus
Developing in a patient with chronic discoid lupus erythematosus of long duration.

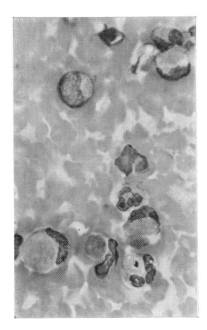

604 Lupus erythematosus cells
Smear from buffy coat stained by Giemsa technique.

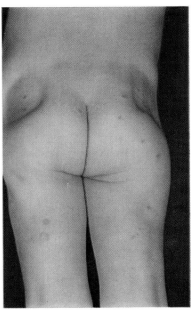

605 Lipodystrophy
Marked atrophy of upper outer gluteal areas following insulin injection.

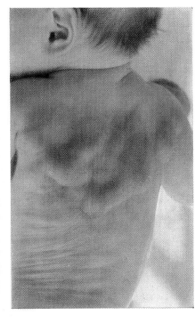

606 Adiponecrosis subcutanea neonatorum
Livid discoloration of the skin with circumscribed areas of rubbery hardening of subcutaneous fat.

Metabolic Skin Diseases

Xanthelasma palpebrarum

This common disorder appears in adult life, forming soft, yellow, flat plaques on the eyelids, predominantly on the medial portion of the upper lids. In about 50 per cent of patients with xanthelasma, serum cholesterol levels are elevated.

Hypercholesteremic xanthomatosis

Another type of essential xanthomatosis (THANNHAUSER) is *primary familial essential hypercholesteremic xanthomatosis*, a disease presumably related to increased cholesterol synthesis. Serum cholesterol and phospholipids are elevated. The serum is clear. The clinical picture is dominated by large, yellow, tuberous xanthomas on the elbows, knees, and extensor surfaces of the hands and feet, by xanthomas of the tendons, and by xanthelasmas.

Secondary forms of hypercholesteremic xanthomas with similar cutaneous symptoms are seen in association with hypothyroidism and certain liver diseases (biliary cirrhosis).

Hyperlipemic xanthomatosis

According to THANNHAUSER, primary idiopathic familial hyperlipemias of adults and the juvenile form with hepatosplenomegaly (BÜRGER-GRÜTZ) belong to the group of hyperlipemic xanthomatoses. In contrast to hypercholesteremic xanthomatosis, which shows a clear serum, the serum in hyperlipemic xanthomatosis is milky. The skin changes consist of small yellowish, disseminated papules on the elbows, knees, gluteal areas, and other parts of the integument. Xanthelasmas of the eyelids are absent.

Secondary hyperlipemias (e.g., in severe forms of diabetes mellitus, nephrosis, or pancreatitis) also may cause skin xanthomas.

The prognosis of hyperlipemic xanthomatosis is favorable inasmuch as it is more readily controlled by a rigid low-fat, cholesterol-free diet.

Necrobiosis lipoidica diabeticorum (URBACH)

This disease is not confined exclusively to diabetics, although it may precede the appearance of diabetes mellitus by many years. It may occur at any age, more frequently in women than in men, usually involving the anterior surfaces of the lower legs.

The characteristic plaque is sharply defined, with an atrophic yellowish center and a bluish-violet peripheral zone; the surface is waxy and slightly telangiectatic. These skin changes evolve from inflammatory vascular processes (lipid deposits in necrobiotic collagen).

Hand-Schüller-Christian Syndrome

The principal symptoms of this etiologically obscure lipid reticulo-endotheliosis are defects in membranous bones (skull), diabetes insipidus, and exophthalmos; occasionally, small papular, yellowish to dark brown, symmetrically disseminated lesions are seen on the head, trunk, and antecubital areas. Children and adolescents are most frequently affected. The disease is often fatal.

Nevoxanthoendothelioma (McDONAGH)

Groups of yellowish or brownish papules or nodules, mostly on the extensor surfaces and on the scalp or neck of infants, are characteristic of this disease. The lesions are lipid-storing histiocytomas, which have a tendency to regress spontaneously in later years. Blood lipid levels are normal.

Lichen amyloidosus

Primary localized cutaneous amyloidoses are rare. The uniform translucent, itching, lichenoid papules are usually located on the extensor surfaces of the lower legs, often in the form of infiltrated moniliform plaques.

Localized pretibial myxedema

Occasionally intercellular accumulation of mucin, distributed symmetrically over the extensor surfaces of the lower legs and the dorsa of the feet, occurs in hyperthyroidism. The plaque-like lesions are yellowish to reddish-brown; the follicular openings are dilated (peau d'orange surface). Marked exophthalmos is usually present simultaneously. The condition also occurs after thyroidectomy.

Calcinosis

Metabolic calcinoses are usually associated with certain dermatoses, or are seen following skin trauma. The calcium deposits occur mainly in the skin, preferably on the extensor aspects of the extremities, the fingers, and the toes. Some dermatoses associated with calcinosis cutis are scleroderma, dermatomyositis, RAYNAUD's disease, and poikiloderma. Rarely, diseases with increased blood calcium levels (e. g., hypervitaminosis D, parathyroid tumors, osteomyelitis, bone tumors) may also cause cutaneous calcinosis.

Gout

Tophi (deposits of sodium urate crystals) usually occur in the form of waxy nodules on the rims of the ears and near the distal points of the extremities. They are pathognomonic of chronic gout, a familial disturbance of nucleic acid metabolism, inherited as a dominant trait occurring primarily in men. The nodules may ulcerate and discharge chalky white material.

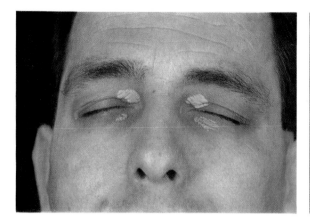

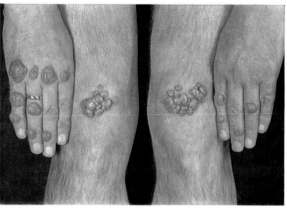

607   Xanthelasma palpebrarum

Flat, soft, yellow plaques of the medial portion of the upper and lower lids.

608   Idiopathic hyperlipemic xanthomatosis

Large, yellow, tuberous xanthomas of the knees and hands. These lesions are more common in hypercholesteremic xanthomatosis.

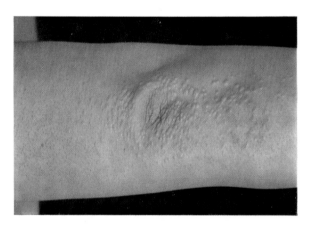

609

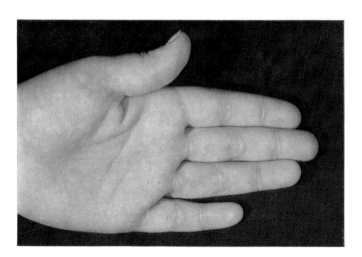

610

609 and **610   Idiopathic hyperlipemic xanthomatosis**

Small, yellow, papular xanthomas of the elbow, with yellowish infiltration of palmar and digital creases.

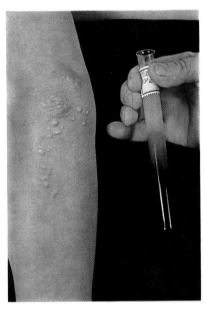

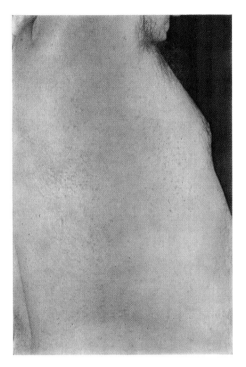

611 Idiopathic hyperlipemic xanthomatosis

Disseminated, small, yellowish papules on the elbows. In contrast to hypercholesteremic xanthomatosis, the blood serum is milky.

612 Secondary hyperlipemic xanthomatosis

Small papular xanthomas in a patient with diabetes mellitus.

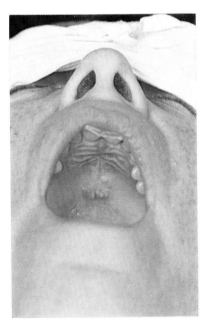

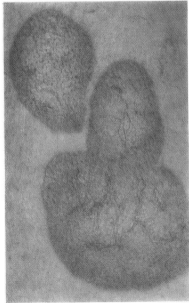

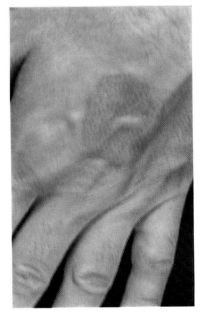

613 Xanthomas

Xanthomatous lesions on the hard and soft palate.

614 Necrobiosis lipoidica diabeticorum

Sharply marginated, yellowish-brown, atrophic plaques on the lower leg with erythematous periphery and central telangiectases.

615 Necrobiosis lipoidica diabeticorum

Circumscribed yellowish-red infiltration with early atrophic changes of the dorsum of the hand.

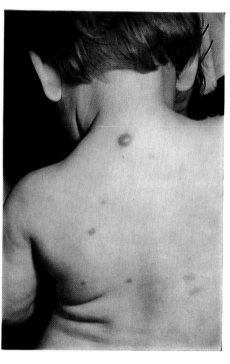

616   Hand-Schüller-Christian syndrome

Disseminated nonspecific, reddish-brown papular skin lesions with bone defects (map-like skull) and diabetes insipidus.

617   Nevoxanthoendothelioma

Multiple yellowish-red and brownish papules and nodules on the back of a child.

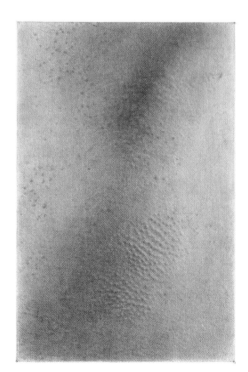

618   Follicular mucinosis

Alopecia mucinosa with pinhead-sized isolated follicular papules.

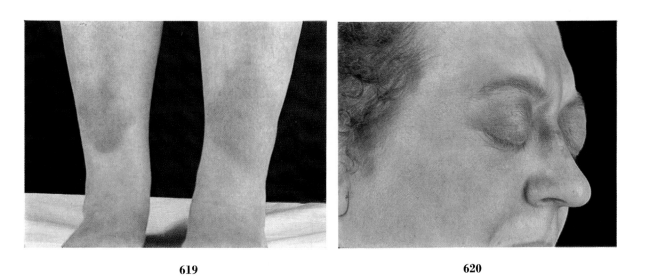

619   **620**

619 and 620   Localized pretibial myxedema

Symmetrical, infiltrated, reddish-brown plaques on the extensor surface of the lower legs with dilated follicular openings (peau d'orange skin) in hyperthyroid patient with marked exophthalmos.

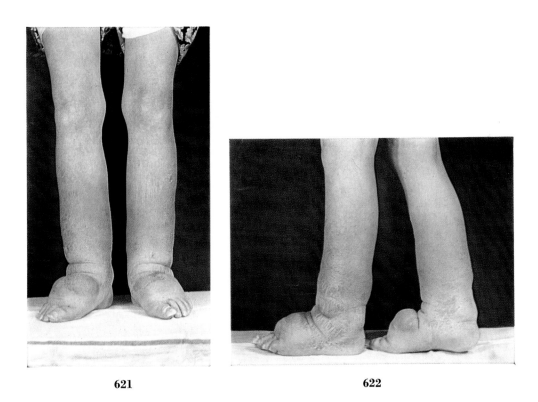

621   **622**

621 and 622   Localized pretibial myxedema

Massive edema of the lower legs resembling elephantiasis, following treatment of hyperthyroidism.

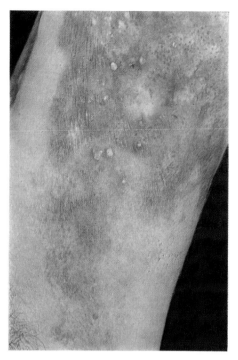

623 Calcinosis cutis
Yellowish-white hard calcium deposits secondary to skin changes of dermatomyositis.

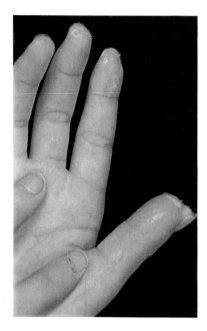

624 Calcinosis cutis
Small calcium deposits of distal phalanges in sclerodactylia.

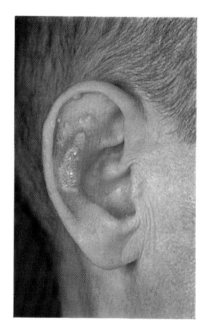

625

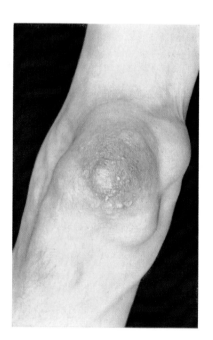

626

625 and **626** **Gout**
Waxy nodules (tophi) of the ear and elbow.

Photodermatoses

All skin changes classified as photodermatoses are induced by exposure to sunlight, and heal when sunlight is eliminated. Ultraviolet rays ranging in wave lengths from 280 mμ to 400 mμ, and visible rays varying from 400 mμ to 760 mμ, are responsible for these changes. A common dermatosis produced by overexposure to sunlight is *dermatitis solaris,* or sunburn. *Phototoxic* substances (oil of bergamot, cumarin — containing essential oils) increase light sensitivity and thus lead to pathologic changes, such as BERLOQUE *dermatitis* and *dermatitis pratensis* (grass dermatitis) or *phytophotodermatitis.* These reactions can be elicited in most persons.

Photoallergic substances (phenothiazines, sulfonamides, demethylchlortetracycline, clearing agents, p-amino-salicylic acid) induce erythema and bulla formation in light-exposed skin areas of sensitized subjects. An antigen-antibody mechanism is operative in this type of reaction.

Chronic polymorphous light eruptions
(HAXTHAUSEN)

The clinical picture of chronic polymorphous light eruptions is varied, comprising papular and eczematous as well as temporary erythematous eruptions with edematous infiltration and lupus erythematosus-like patches. The diagnosis is confirmed by localization of the eruptions in light-exposed areas, remission during fall and winter, and phototests with various light sources after elimination of the erythematogenic range (below 320 mμ) with special filters. Three types of this condition have been described: eczematous, lupus, erythematosus-like, and erythematous light eruption (WULF). Indolylacrylic acid can be demonstrated in the urine.

Solar urticaria (MERKLEN)

Familial incidence of urticaria in exposed areas following brief exposure to sunlight, occasionally associated with malaise and syncope, has been described in the literature. An antigen-antibody mechanism is believed to be the pathogenetic basis of this reaction.

Solar dermatosis of spring (BURCKHARDT)

In early spring, children and adolescents may develop erythema, bullae, and papules, usually on the rims of the ears, more rarely on the dorsa of the hands and fingers. Sunlight is a proved etiologic factor in this rare condition; it is possible that cold is also important.

Actinic cheilitis
(Summer cheilitis; MARCHIONINI)

During the hot season, UV-radiation may produce inflammatory erythema, blistering, and crust formation on the lower lip.

Cutaneous porphyrias

Congenital porphyria
(Erythropoietic porphyria; GÜNTHER)

This very rare disease, probably transmitted as a mendelian recessive trait more common in boys than in girls, usually manifests itself soon after birth. Burgundy-red to brown discoloration of the urine may be the first visible sign of the disease. Significant amounts of porphyrin, predominantly uroporphyrin I and coproporphyrin I, but no porphobilinogen are excreted in the urine. Uroporphyrin I, a photosensitizer, is responsible for the rapidly progressive course of the illness which manifests itself clinically as a photodermatosis. In light-exposed areas of the skin, small itching necroses surrounded by erythema appear, develop into vesicles and hemorrhagic blisters (*hydroa aestivale*) and eventually lead to atrophy, ulceration, scarring, hyperpigmentation, and milia; severe mutilations of the ear, nose, eyelids, and fingers (*hydroa vacciniforme*) may result. Associated symptoms are anemia, splenomegaly, photophobia, conjunctivitis, keratitis, and erythrodontia. Urinary excretion of porphyrin usually is grossly visible, but smaller amounts may be visualized under WOOD's light (reddish fluorescence). Some of the red blood cells also fluoresce under WOOD's light owing to their high content of uroporphyrin I and coroporphyrin I. The probable cause of this inborn error of metabolism is the lack of a specific enzyme (isomerase).

Porphyria cutanea tarda (WALDENSTRÖM)
(Chronic hepatic porphyria [WATSON])

WALDENSTRÖM differentiated between hereditary and symptomatic porphyria cutanea tarda. Some authors attribute the disease to hepatic damage (alcohol) in association with genetic factors. Others assume a disturbance in porphyrin metabolism on the basis of hepatic impairment due to alcohol, arsenic, barbiturates, or hepatitis. The metabolic defect is believed to be due to decarboxylase deficiency of the liver cell.

Porphyria cutanea tarda is one of the most common forms of cutaneous porphyria, and is usually seen in males with chronic liver damage in the 40 to 60 age group. Short solar exposure or slight traumatization may produce small vesicles or bullae which eventually may lead to erosions, crusts, milia, atrophy, flat scars, hypo- or hyperpigmentation, and hypertrichosis. Urinary porphyrin levels are increased.

Xeroderma pigmentosum (KAPOSI)

Exposure to sunlight initially produces erythema and scaling, later hyperpigmented spots, and eventually atrophic scars and telangiectases similar to those seen in chronic radiodermatitis. The disease may have its onset in early infancy. Face, neck, upper chest, hands, and forearms are involved. As in chronic radiodermatitis, keratoses and papillomas with a tendency to malignant degeneration (usually carcinomatous) may develop. The disease is inherited as a recessive gene. Patients in whom it becomes manifest at an early age rarely survive adolescence.

Hartnup Syndrome (DENT)

This syndrome (named after the HARTNUP family) is characterized by a pellagroid dermatitis following exposure to light, intermittent cerebellar ataxia, aminoaciduria (cysteine, cystine, glycine, serine, glutamine, asparagine, histidine), and urinary excretion of indolacetic acid, indoxyl sulfate, and indolylacetylglutamic acid. KIMMIG was the first author to demonstrate indolylacrylic acid in the urine of patients with HARTNUP syndrome. This acid is an endogenous photosensitizing agent which has been demonstrated in polymorphous photodermatoses, dermatitis solaris, subacute lupus erythematosus, and following phenothiazine medication. HARTNUP syndrome is based on a disturbance in tryptophane metabolism, and is inherited as a recessive condition.

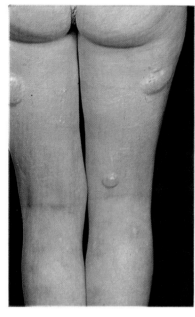

627 Acute solar dermatitis
Severe erythema and large bullae
of thighs (sunburn).

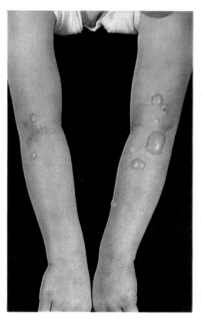

628 Toxic photodermatitis
Bullous reaction due to coal tar
and sunlight.

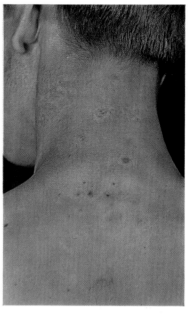

**629 Toxic photodermatitis of
the neck**
Due to chlorinated anthracene
oil (coal tar fraction).

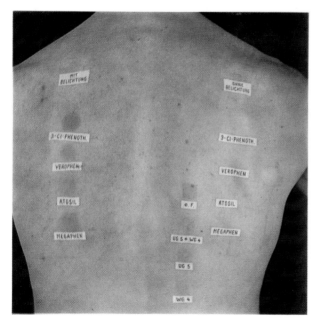

630 Allergic photodermatitis
Due to phenothiazine derivative. Erythema of the face
and neck. Patch tests negative without light exposure
(right side), positive with light exposure (left side).

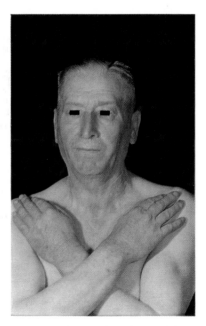

631 Allergic photodermatitis
Due to oral antidiabetic drug
(tolbutamide).

208

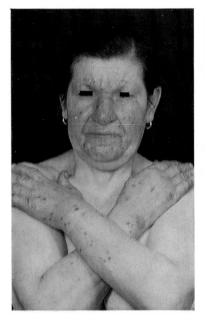

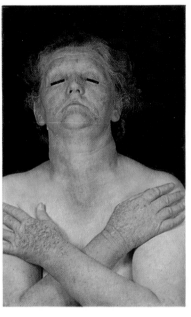

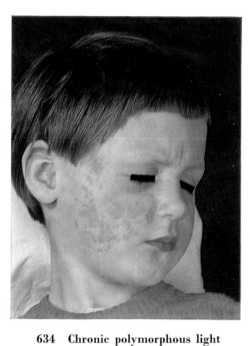

632 Chronic polymorphous light eruption

Eczematous type with papular lesions, excoriations, and lichenification of the skin.

633 Chronic polymorphous light eruption

Lichenification of the face and hands. Typically, the submental area is not affected.

634 Chronic polymorphous light eruption

Erythematous scaling patches resembling lupus erythematosus.

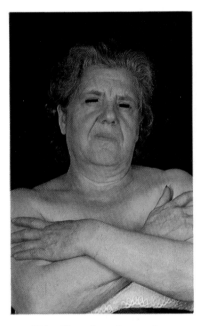

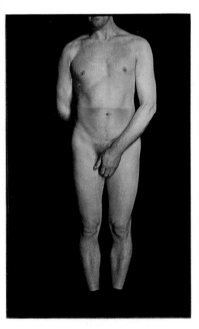

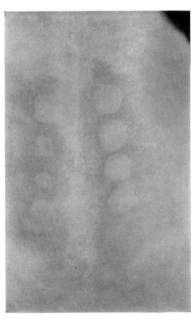

635 Chronic polymorphous light eruption

Erythematous type, resembling protracted sunburn.

636 Solar urticaria (familial type)

Urticarial wheals in light exposed areas.

637 Solar urticaria

Small areas exposed to different doses of sunlight show wheals with red flares.

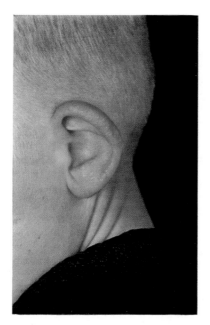

638 **Solar dermatosis of spring** (BURCKHARDT)
Edema and vesiculation on the ear
lobe of a young child.

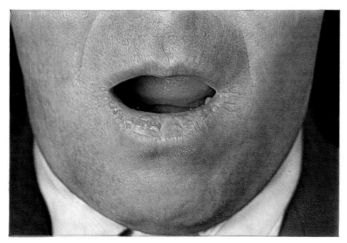

639 **Actinic cheilitis**
Erythema, edema, and scaling of the lower lip.

641 and **642** **Congenital (erythropoietic) porphyria**
Erythrodontia and severe necroses of the hands and face.

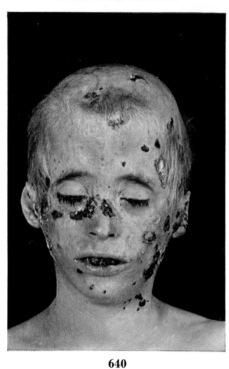

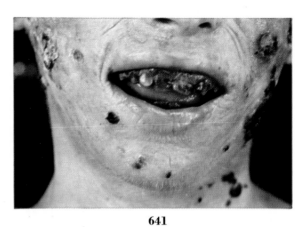

641

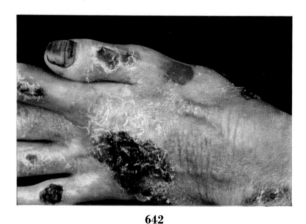

640

642

640 **Congenital (erythropoietic) porphyria (hydroa vacciniforme).** Hemorrhagic blisters, crusts, necroses, and scars in areas of face exposed to light, associated with systemic symptoms.

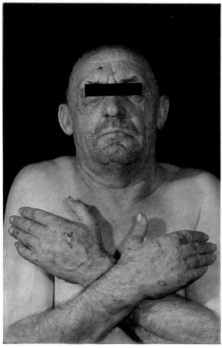

643 **Porphyria cutanea tarda**
Hepatic porphyria with crusted lesions of the face and hands.

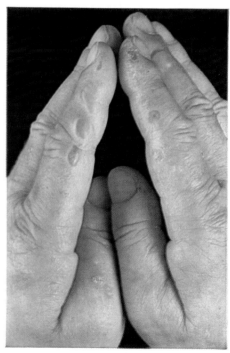

644 **Porphyria cutanea tarda**
Vesicles, crusts, and shallow scars.

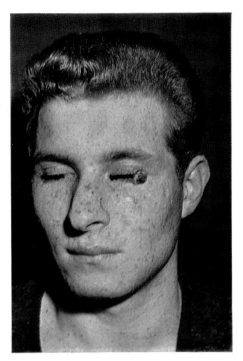

645   Xeroderma pigmentosum
Typical atrophic skin changes resembling chronic radiodermatitis. Squamous cell carcinoma on the left lower
eyelid.

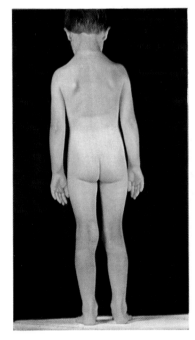

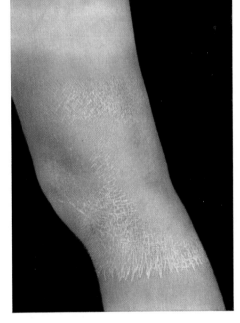

646   **647**

646 and **647**   HARTNUP **syndrome**
Familial pellagroid dermatitis of exposed skin areas.

Reactions to Physical and Chemical Agents

Mechanical injury including pressure, friction, and rubbing may, under certain conditions, provoke pigmentation, blistering, and hyperkeratoses of the skin. Constant pressure may lead to local anemia and necrosis of the skin (decubitus).

Thermal burns are caused by open flame, hot vapors, molten metals, or radiant heat; *scalds* are caused by hot liquids. First-degree burns or scalds are characterized by erythema; second-degree injuries by blister formation; and third-degree injuries by necrosis. Determination of the depth and extent of the injury is prognostically significant. *Frostbite* starts at the acra. First-degree frostbite leads to vasoconstriction, sometimes to the point of ischemia. Brief and fairly superficial exposure to cold results in erythema and paresthesia followed by complete recovery. Longer and deeper exposure leads to blister formation (second-degree frostbite) or necrosis (third-degree frostbite).

Chemical burns due to alkalis and certain acids are of special importance in the field of occupational dermatoses. Chromic acid causes circumscribed ulceration of the skin. Arsenical compounds may produce eczema and ulceration. Bleaching of hair with undiluted peroxide solution frequently results in damage to the scalp. Indiscriminate use of phenol as a disinfectant or caustic agent also may cause considerable damage.

In addition to accidental injuries, skin damage is sometimes produced deliberately by certain patients with the aid of chemical agents. A popular and easily available agent for the production of such *artefacts* is glacial acetic acid (50 to 80 per cent acetic acid).

Electrical injuries of the skin may be produced with any electrical device having a voltage of 60 V or more. Depending on the conditions of the exposure, localized or extensive burns may result.

Ionizing radiation (x-rays, grenz rays, radium, radiocobalt, thorium X) may produce varying degrees of *radiodermatitis*, depending on the dosage administered; the latent period may range from 1 to 12 days.

Acute radiodermatitis

First-degree radiodermatitis is characterized by erythema and edema, followed by patchy hyperpigmentation, temporary alopecia, and transient reduction of sebum production. A second-degree injury produces erythema, edema, vesiculation, irreversible loss of nails and hair, and diminished sebaceous gland activity. Third-degree radiodermatitis leads to acute roentgen ulcer in addition to the skin changes described above.

Chronic radiodermatitis

This can be caused by repeated small exposures or single large doses of ionizing radiation that initially were followed by first- to third-degree acute radiodermatitis. Atrophy, telangiectasia, depigmentation or hyperpigmentation, permanent alopecia, shedding of nails, and keratotic changes are seen after varying periods of time.

Late complications of chronic radiodermatitis are *chronic radiation ulcer* and *x-ray cancer* (both basal cell epithelioma and prickle cell carcinoma). These may occur as late as 10 to 20 years after the original damage.

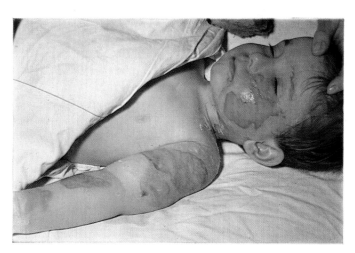

648

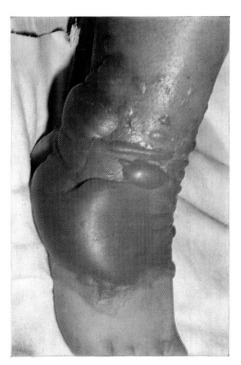

649

648 and **649**   **Second-degree scalds**
Large blisters, erosions, and superficial ulcers caused by hot water.

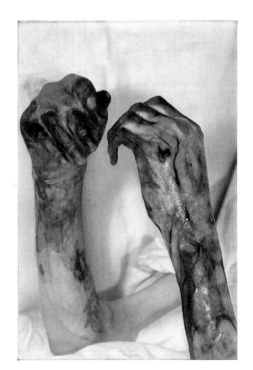

650   **Third-degree burn**
With large necrotic areas.

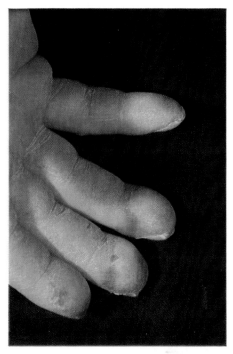

651   **Second-degree frostbite**
Blister formation on fingertips.

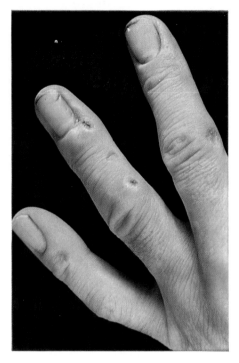

652 Chemical burn
Small ulcers due to chromic acid
compound.

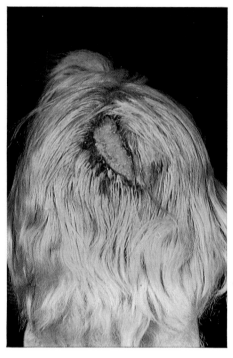

653 Chemical burn
Large ulceration of the scalp due to
peroxide treatment.

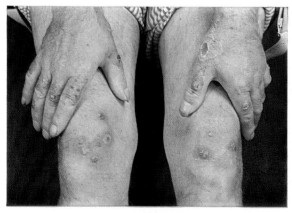

654 Chemical burn
Due to arsenic compound.

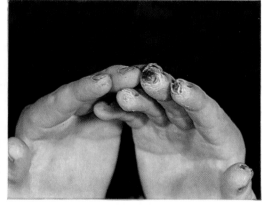

655 Chemical burn
Due to hydrofluoric acid.

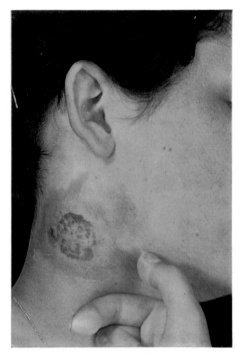

656 Factitial ulcer

Chemical burn due to glacial acetic acid. Erythema and superficial ulceration of the neck; bullae of the thumb and index finger.

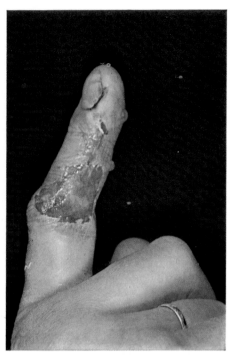

657 Chemical burn

Caused by an antimycotic agent containing phenol.

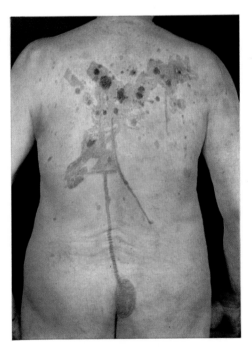

658 Chemical burn

Due to careless treatment of seborrheic keratoses with phenol.

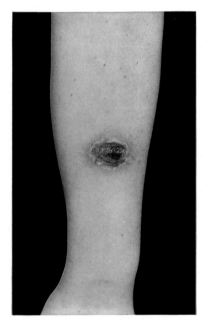

659 Factitial dermatitis

Chemical burn due to hydrochloric acid (self-inflicted).

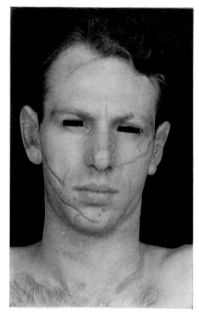

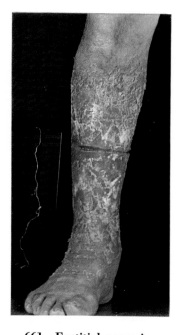

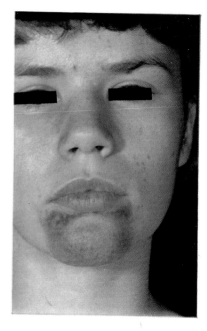

660 Factitial dermatitis
Linear chemical burns due to an acid.

661 Factitial necrosis
Patient had tied the string pictured at left around his lower leg, causing the skin to become necrotic. The string was so far ingrown that it almost escaped detection.

662 Factitial hematoma
Self-inflicted by suction.

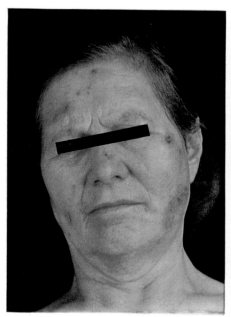

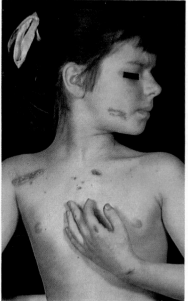

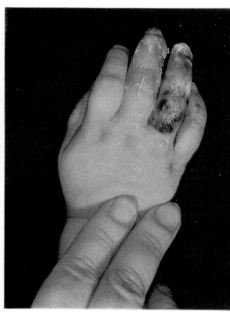

663 Neurotic excoriations
Patient had delusions of parasitosis.

664

665

664 and **665 Electrical injury.** Necrotic lesions caused by electric current.

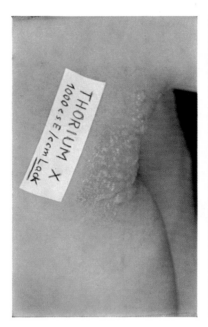

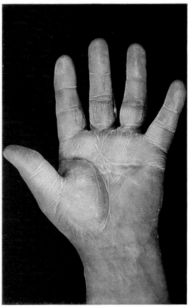

666　Acute radiodermatitis

Erythematovesicular reaction
caused by thorium X lacquer.

667　Acute radiodermatitis

Severe bullous reaction following
shortly after excessive dosage
of x-rays.

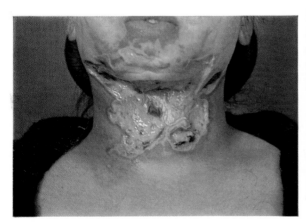

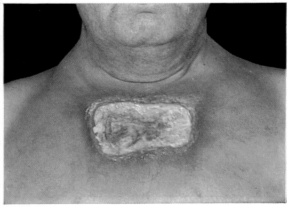

668　X-ray ulcer

Following excessive dosage of x-rays for hypertrichosis.

669　X-ray ulcer

Following massive irradiation of a retrosternal
tumor.

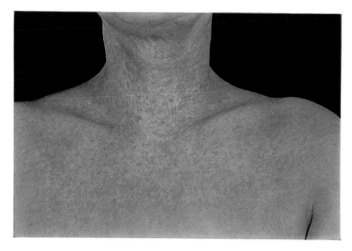

670   Chronic radiodermatitis

Due to frequent x-ray treatments of atopic dermatitis. Atrophy, pigment changes, telangiectases, hair loss, and fibrotic and keratotic changes.

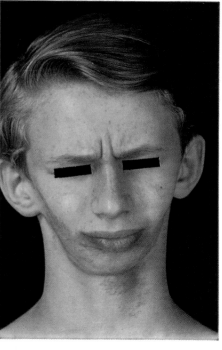

671   Chronic radiodermatitis

Nevus flammeus treated with x-rays during first year of life. The residual nevus is now complicated by a chronic radiodermatitis and atrophy of the mandible.

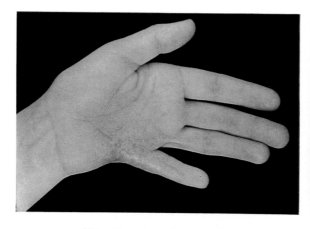

672   Chronic radiodermatitis

Hemangioma irradiated with radium during the first year of life. Chronic radiodermatitis and dystrophy of the fifth digit.

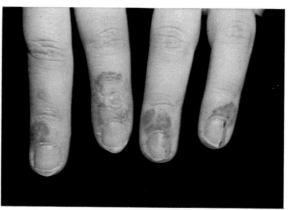

673   Chronic radiodermatitis

Erythematous sclerotic changes due to excessive x-ray treatment of warts.

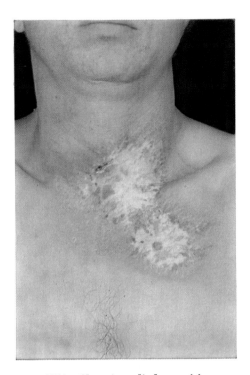

674 Chronic radiodermatitis

White sclerotic and atrophic areas with
marked telangiectasia and small ulcerations due to overdosage of x-rays in a
diagnostic attempt to localize metal
particles.

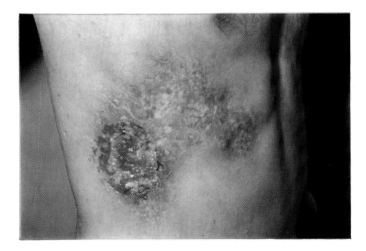

675 Chronic radiodermatitis

Large chronic radiation ulcer, hyperpigmentation and
depigmentation, telangiectasia and sclerosis following excessive x-ray treatment of a hemangioma.

Leukemias and Lymphomas

Uncontrolled proliferation of the cells of the hemopoietic system may lead to appearance of pathological cells in the peripheral blood and, occasionally, in the skin. More frequently, however, the pathological process originates in and remains confined to the skin. Proliferation of immature forms of white blood cells produces myeloid or lymphoid leukemia; that of immature red blood cells, erythroblastoses; and that of cells of the reticuloendothelial system, reticuloses.

While many European textbooks classify both mycosis fungoides and HODGKIN's disease as systemic granulomatoses, most American authors regard mycosis fungoides as a lymphoma. *Mycosis fungoides* originates in the skin and usually remains confined to the integument for a long period of time. HODGKIN's *disease* rarely manifests itself with specific infiltrates of the skin, and even less often originates in the skin. Both diseases are severe systemic disorders, histologically characterized predominantly by chronic granulomatous inflammation with more or less marked proliferation of reticulohistiocytic elements.

Leukemia cutis

Chronic myeloid leukemia

Cutaneous manifestations of myeloid leukemia are extremely rare, while those of lymphatic leukemia are seen somewhat more frequently. Papular eruptions, purpura, hemorrhagic nodules of the mucous membranes, solitary ulcerating skin tumors, priapism, and splenomegaly are all signs suggestive of chronic myeloid leukemia.

Chronic lymphatic leukemia

This condition may be characterized by persistent pruritus, polymorphous erythematous eruptions, bullae, vegetating lesions, bluish-red painless nodules or tumors located on prominent areas of the face (leonine facies), with virtually no tendency to regression but a strong tendency to ulcerative degeneration. Diagnosis is made by histologic examination of the skin lesions, bone marrow smear, and peripheral blood count.

Reticulosis cutis

This disease originates in the skin, manifesting a disturbance of the ubiquitous, plurifunctional, and polyvalent reticuloendothelial system. The histologically *monomorphous type* produces large, nodular, plate-like, or small papular or nodular exanthematous or erythrodermic skin lesions. Monocytoid cells may appear in the peripheral blood. The most common *polymorphous reticulosis* is urticaria pigmentosa.

Urticaria pigmentosa (Mastocytoma)

Urticaria pigmentosa (mastocytoma) was first described by Nettleship. This mast cell reticulosis of the skin may appear in infancy, puberty, or at a later age. Round or oval, light-to-dark-brown maculopapular lesions measuring 1 to 25 mm. in diameter are seen, especially on the trunk and the proximal portions of the extremities. Friction produces a wheal confined to the site of mechanical irritation — a significant diagnostic sign. Occasionally, this may lead to bulla formation (*bullous urticaria pigmentosa*). Large nodular forms of mast cell reticulosis have been observed also.

The disease shows a tendency toward slow spontaneous regression. Rarely, it may lead to fatal *mast cell leukemia*.

Lymphadenosis benigna cutis (BÄFVERSTEDT) (Lymphocytoma)

This secondary, reversible reticulosis of the skin is believed to be caused by an infectious agent. The preferred site of the large nodular lymphocytoma is the ear lobe.

Granuloma faciale eosinophilicum (WIGLEY)

Preferred areas of this entity, which is not related to eosinophilic granuloma of bone, are the cheeks, temples, and nose. The lesions are sharply defined, soft, round or polycyclic, with a more or less irregular surface, and of red, bluish-red, or yellowish-brown color. The etiology of the disorder is unknown.

Mycosis fungoides (d'ALIBERT-BAZIN)

The cause of mycosis fungoides is unknown. Death may occur within six months; many patients survive 5 to 20 years, however. The disease usually has its onset in the second half of life and may manifest itself in three different forms: the *classic progressive type* (D'ALIBERT-BAZIN), the *erythrodermic type* (HALLOPEAU-BESNIER, "l'homme rouge"), and the *"d'emblée"* type (VIDAL-BROCQ), which begins with tumors.

The *initial stage* of *classic mycosis fungoides* is characterized by nonspecific, pruritic, evanescent urticarial patches, eczematous lesions, psoriasiform or parapsoriatic eruptions, and — occasionally — vesicular changes (erythematous, premycotic or prefungoid stage).

The *second stage* shows flat and nodular infiltrations (plaque stage); the *third*, typical mycotic tumors (tumor stage).

In the *"d'emblée" type*, mycotic tumors arise from normal skin or mucous membranes, without visible preceding skin changes.

The *erythrodermic type* is a generalized exfoliative dermatitis associated with general lymphadenopathy.

Hodgkin's disease (Lymphogranulomatosis)

Various cutaneous changes may occur in HODGKIN's disease. An important symptom, and sometimes one of the earliest, is pruritus. Excoriations, hyperpigmentation, urticarial or papular changes and pruriginous nodules ("prurigo lymphadenique" DUBREUILH) are some of the nonspecific skin manifestations. Specific changes are plate-like infiltrates and necrotizing brownish-red nodules originating in the skin; infiltrations extending into the skin in contiguity with lymph nodes; acquired ichthyosis; and the large purplish, rapidly ulcerating tumors characteristic of that form of malignant lymphogranulomatosis that originates primarily in the skin.

Systemic symptoms of HODGKIN's disease are unilateral cervical lymphadenopathy, intermittent fever (PEL-EBSTEIN type), anemia, eosinophilia, intolerance to alcohol, and progressive involvement of lymph nodes.

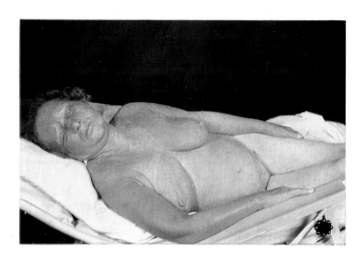

676 Chronic myeloid leukemia
Associated with erythroderma and generalized pruritus.

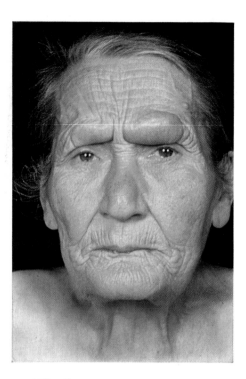

677 Chronic lymphatic leukemia
Reddish-blue, painless, tumorous infiltrates of the eyebrow region.

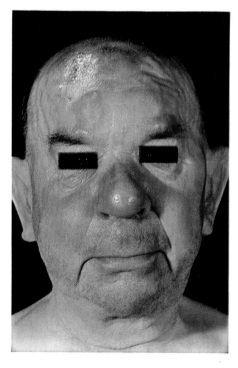

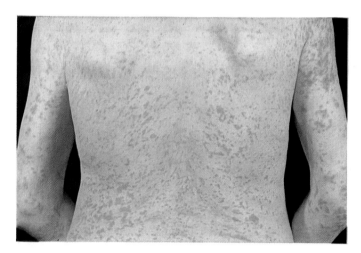

679 Chronic lymphatic leukemia
Disseminated papular infiltrates of the back and extremities with marked pruritus.

678 Chronic lymphatic leukemia. Diffuse and nodular infiltrates of prominent areas of the face (leonine facies).

678

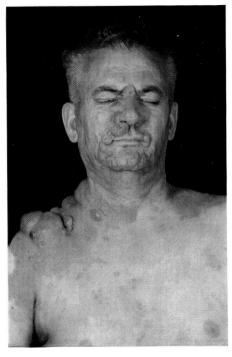

680   Reticulosis cutis
With large nodular and plate-like lesions (histologically monomorphous type).

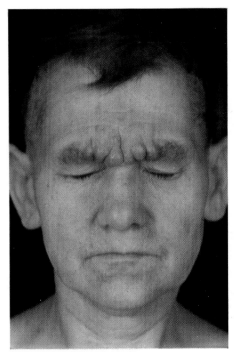

681   Reticulosis cutis
With large nodular lesions of the face (histologically monomorphous type).

682   Reticulosis cutis
With small nodules and scaling papules (histologically monomorphous type).

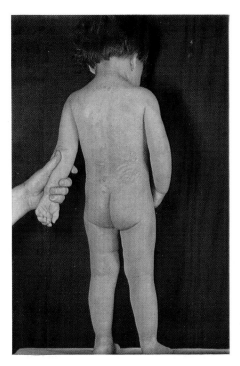

683   Urticaria pigmentosa
Diffuse cutaneous mastocytomas with typical urticarial reaction following friction of lesions on the mid-back.

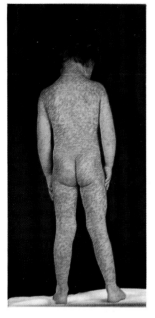
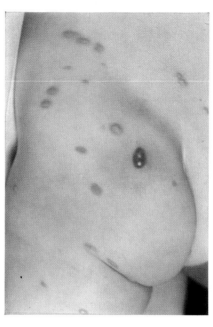
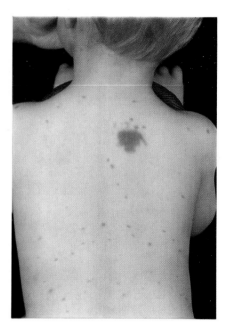

684 Urticaria pigmentosa
Generalized brownish
maculopapular lesions.

685 Urticaria pigmentosa
Characteristic round to oval reddish-
brown nodules and large bulla.

686 Urticaria pigmentosa
Discrete and plaque-like mastocytomas of upper back.

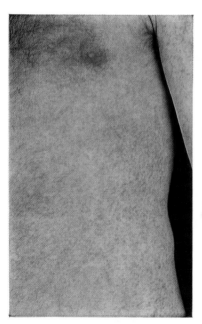
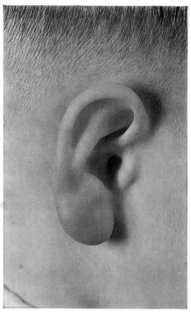
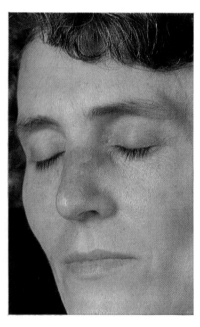

687 Urticaria pigmentosa
Onset at adult age.

688 Lymphadenosis benigna cutis
Large, red, nodular lymphocytoma in typical localization.

689 Lymphadenosis benigna cutis
Circumscribed reddish infiltration
of the nose.

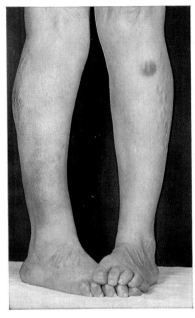

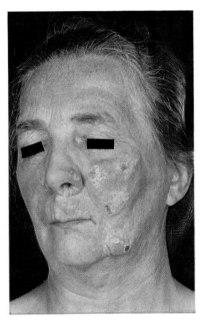

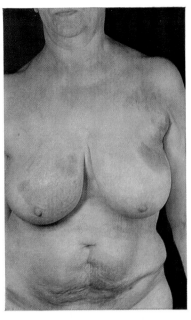

690 Lymphocytoma

Tumor below the left knee associated with acrodermatitis chronica atrophicans HERXHEIMER.

691 Granuloma faciale eosinophilicum

Bluish-red, soft, scaling infiltration of the left cheek and the nose.

692 Mycosis fungoides, plaque stage

Circumscribed, flat, pruritic, infiltrated patches.

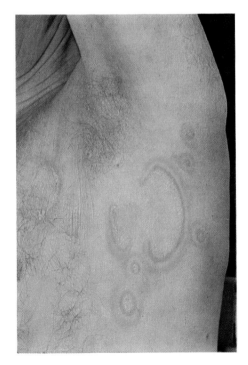

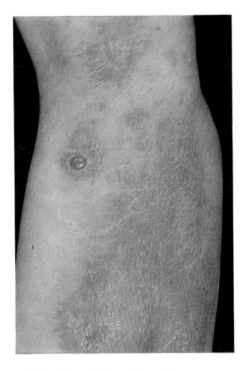

693 Mycosis fungoides, plaque stage

Bizarre circinate and polycyclic infiltrations with erythematous border.

694 Mycosis fungoides, plaque stage

Pruritic, erythematosquamous, firm infiltrations with blister formation.

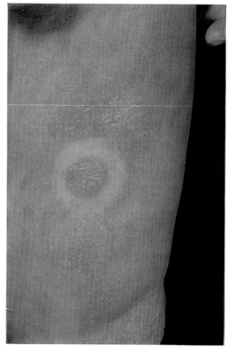

695 Mycosis fungoides, plaque stage

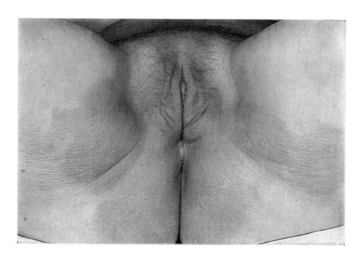

696 Mycosis fungoides, plaque stage
Circumscribed pruritic infiltration of
anogenital region.

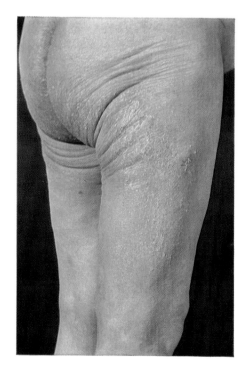

697 Mycosis fungoides, plaque stage. Large, violaceous-red,
scaling infiltrations of the thighs and gluteal area.

698 Erythrodermic mycosis fungoides (l'homme rouge)
Generalized exfoliative dermatitis with lymphadenopathy.

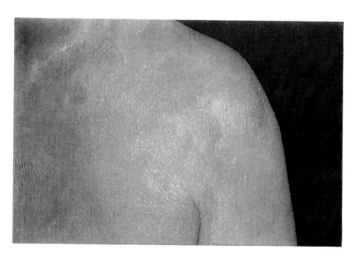

697

698

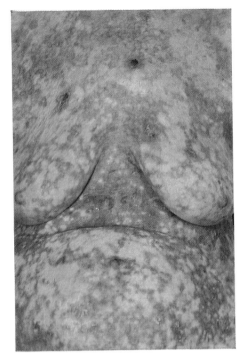

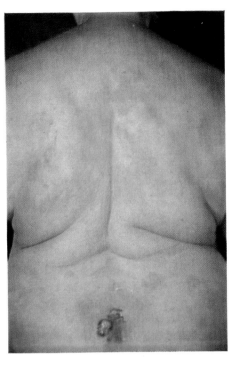

699   Mycosis fungoides
Developing in preexisting parapsoriasis variegata.

700   Mycosis fungoides
Developing in preexisting parapsoriasis en plaques.

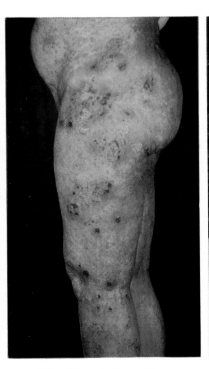

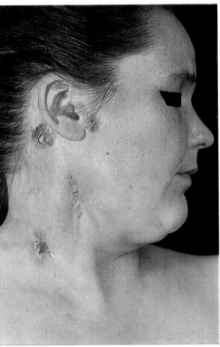

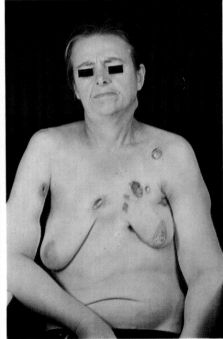

701   Mycosis fungoides, tumor stage
Numerous nodular and tumorous infiltrations with partial ulceration.

702

703

702 and 703   Hodgkin's disease (lymphogranulomatosis)
Specific brownish-red necrotizing lesions involving the skin from underlying specific foci.

Congenital Abnormalities of the Skin

Congenital abnormalities, i.e., developmental disturbances confined to a certain part of the organism, may be genetically determined and thus hereditary, or may develop accidentally during intrauterine life.

Aplasia cutis circumscripta

The newborn shows congenital circumscribed ulcerations of the skin which will heal with scarring after several months. The pathogenesis of the disorder is unknown. Hereditary and acquired forms have been observed.

Cutis laxa (D'ALIBERT)

Abnormal elasticity of the skin in circumscribed areas is referred to as cutis laxa or cutis hyperelastica (cf. EHLERS-DANLOS syndrome).

Pterygium colli

Pterygia usually occur on the neck; they also may be found between the fingers and on the bends of the joints. They are often associated with bone and other developmental anomalies (e.g., in BONNEVIE-ULLRICH syndrome).

Branchiogenic fistulas

Congenital branchiogenic fistulas are seen not infrequently, particularly in the preauricular region. Granulomatous inflammatory changes around the fistulous opening (lupoid changes, ulceration) may complicate the diagnosis.

Nevi

On the basis of clinical and practical considerations, this heading includes all circumscribed changes of the skin, whether congenital or appearing later in life, which differ from the surrounding normal skin by abnormal pigmentation or abnormal structure of the epidermis, dermis and vasculature, usually persisting unchanged throughout life. Hereditary factors are important in some instances.

Lentigo (Nevus spilus)

Lentigines are sharply circumscribed smooth dark brown macules, which histologically show hyperpigmentation and increased numbers of clear cells but no nevus cells. *Juvenile lentigines* appear in childhood on all parts of the body. *Senile lentigines* (liver spots) are common in light exposed areas of elderly patients (dorsa of hands, forearms, face).

Melanocytic nevus (Nevus cell nevus)

The essential criterion of these tumors, which are also known as pigmented moles, are nevus cells arranged in groups (modified melanocytes). Melanocytic nevi represent dysontogenetic tumors (hamartomas) possessing a highly differentiated organoid structure (VON ALBERTINI). According to their shape and surface structure, the nevus cell nevi are divided into lentigo-like, papillomatous, verrucous, pigmented and hairy, molluscoid, and hard fibroid moles. The blue nevus of JADASSOHN is rare.

Juvenile melanoma (Spindle cell nevus)

The juvenile melanoma, a very active type of compound nevus (SPITZ), is seen predominantly in the face, and almost exclusively in infants. The prognosis is favorable. Malignant degeneration after puberty has been observed. Because of the presence of pleomorphic spindle cells, these rare tumors are also called spindle cell nevi.

Organic nevi

These are congenital tumors which show an increased number of normal adnexae of the skin, e.g., sebaceous nevi.

Syringoma (Syringocystadenoma)

Syringomas develop from the epithelium of sweat glands. They usually occur on the chest, face, or upper arms of adult women as small, yellowish, soft, discrete nodules.

Vascular nevi

The most common vascular nevus is the *nevus flammeus* (port-wine stain, capillary hemangioma). Others are *nevus araneus* (spider nevus), *nevus vasculosus* (strawberry mark), and *hemangioma cavernosum*.

Occasionally, nevi flammei may be associated with other developmental disturbances. In STURGE-WEBER'S syndrome (encephalotrigeminal angiomatosis) a unilateral nevus flammeus of the upper and middle branches of the trigeminal nerve is associated with glaucoma, epileptic seizures, hemiplegia, and other cerebral disorders.

Klippel-Trénaunay (Parkes-Weber) syndrome
(Osteohypertrophic varicose nevus)

This condition is characterized by a nevus flammeus associated with unilateral partial hypertrophy of skin and bones, and with varicose veins.

Lymphangioma circumscriptum

Groups of deep-seated, skin-colored or yellowish, translucent, thick-walled vesicles (resembling frog's spawn) may be present at birth or appear during the first years of life on the axillae, proximal extremities, scapulae, and mouth. When opened they exude clear odorless lymph. Sometimes the fluid is hemorrhagic. Lymphangiomas may exist in combination with hemangiomas.

230

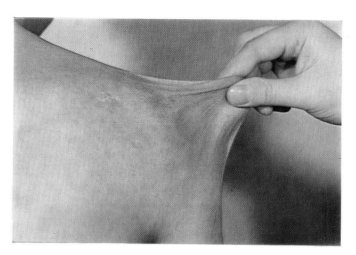

704   Cutis laxa
Isolated lesion on the right shoulder.

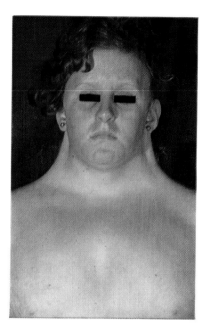

705   Pterygium colli
Widespread   involvement   in   a
young woman.

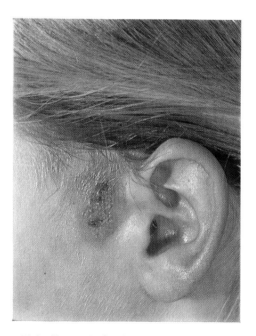

706   Preauricular branchiogenic fistula
Complicated by granulomatous changes
of surrounding skin.

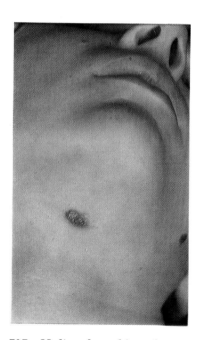

**707   Median branchiogenic cer-
vical fistula**
With brownish, eczematous irritation.

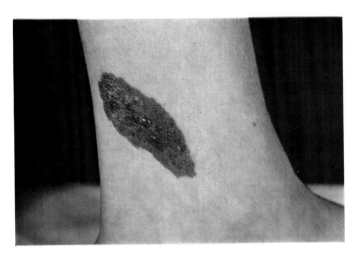

708   Verrucous and pigmented nevus

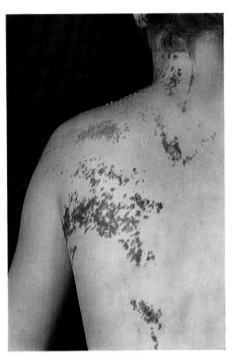

709   Systematized verrucous keratotic nevus

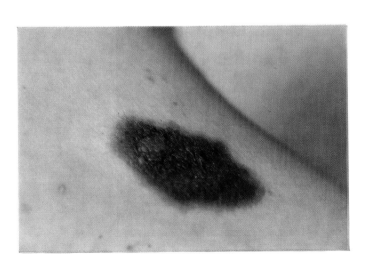

710   Verrucous hairy pigmented nevus

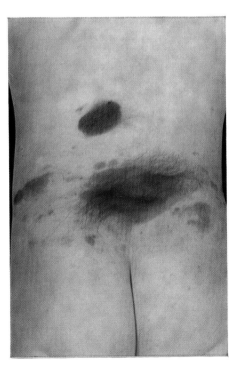

711   Pigmented hairy nevi

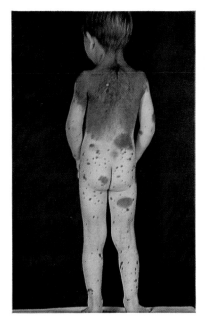

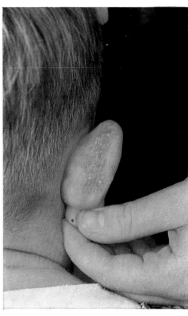

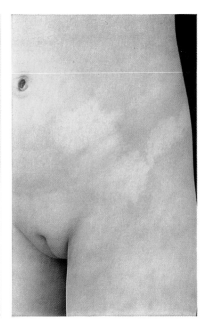

712 Hairy pigmented nevus
Extensive involvement of trunk and extremities.

713 Nevus comedonicus
Circumscribed patch with numerous comedo-like lesions.

714 Nevus achromicus
Absence of pigment in irregular patch with normal surrounding skin.

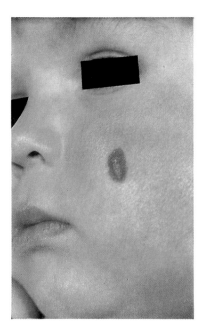

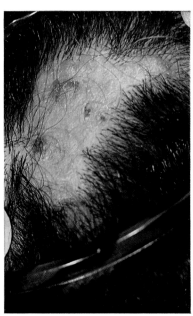

715 Juvenile melanoma (spindle cell nevus)
Reddish, raised, hairless tumor on the cheek of an infant.

716 Nevus sebaceus (JADASSOHN)
Yellowish-red firm plaque with smooth surface and secondary irritation. Present since birth.

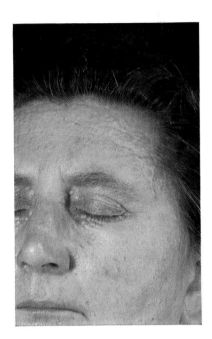

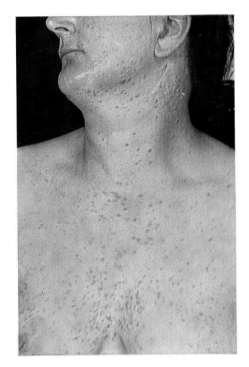

717

718

717 and **718**   **Syringomas**
Numerous discrete, soft, yellowish-red, pinhead-sized nodules on the forehead,
eyelids, face, neck, and upper chest.

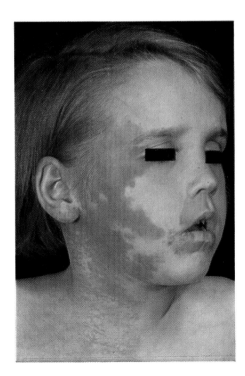

719   Nevus flammeus
Macular, violaceous discoloration with irregular
border on the right side of the face and neck.

720   Nevus flammeus
Irregular, flat, reddish-blue discoloration of the
right cheek and oral mucosa of the lips and gums.

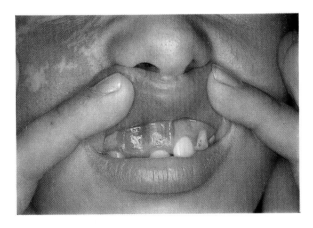

719

720

234

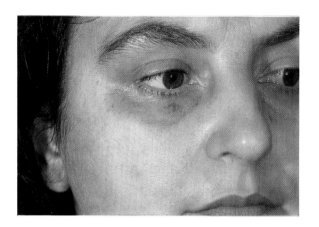

721 Nevus araneus (spider nevus)
With prominent central vessel.

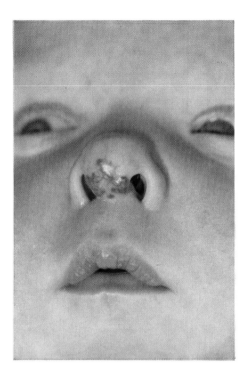

722 Hemangioma cavernosum
Soft, raised, bluish-red nodules involving the nasal septum.

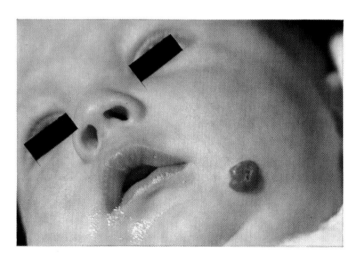

723 Nevus vasculosus (strawberry mark)
Soft, raised, bluish-red tumor with irregular surface and beginning central ulceration.

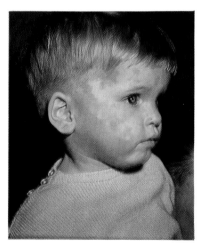

724 Sturge-Weber syndrome
Unilateral nevus flammeus associated with glaucoma and neurological changes.

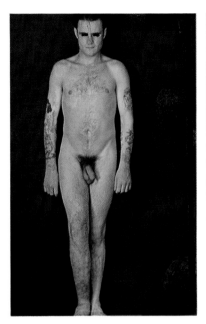

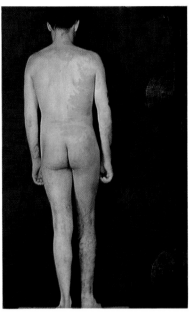

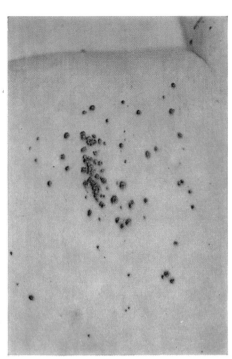

725   **726**

**725 and 726   Klippel-Trénaunay syndrome
(nevus varicosus osteohypertrophicus)**
Widespread unilateral nevus flammeus of the right side with
varicose veins and hypertrophy of the right leg and arm.

727   Lymphangioma circumscriptum
Discrete and grouped, deep-seated,
brownish, thick-walled vesicular lesions.

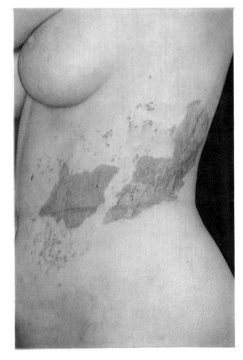

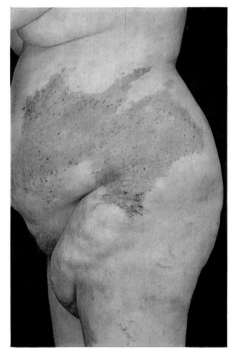

728   Hemangiolymphangioma
In zosteriform distribution on the left
side of the abdomen.

729   Subcutaneous lymphangioma
With circumscribed brownish-bluish
discoloration of the skin surface.

Tumors of the Skin

Benign Tumors

Benign epidermal tumors include *papillomas*, *actinic keratoses* (senile keratoses; occasionally associated with cornu cutaneum), *seborrheic keratoses* (seborrheic warts, verrucae seniles), *keratoacanthomas* (often resembling squamous cell carcinomas), and benign tumors of the skin adnexae. The latter group includes *milia* (white spherical, pinhead-sized cysts, usually occurring in the orbital area or adjacent to scars; especially common in epidermolysis bullosa), *keratinous cysts, mucous cysts, sebaceous cysts, atheromas* (epidermoid or dermoid cysts), *syringomas, cylindromas* (Spiegler tumors; usually in the scalp region of adults). The *calcifying epithelioma of Malherbe*, a solitary tumor situated in the cutis, originates from hair matrix cells which resemble basal cells histologically. *Fibroma pendulum* (molluscum pendulum, acrochordon, skin tag) is a benign dermo-epidermal tumor. Dermal (mesenchymal) tumors include *keloid, fibroma durum*, and other types of fibroma.

Lipomas (hypertrophy of fatty tissue) may occur as solitary or multiple tumors. *Leiomyomas* arise from the arrector muscles of the hair or from the muscles of the blood vessels; these tumors are painful. Another mesenchymal tumor is *granuloma pyogenicum* (granuloma telangiectatum), an eruptive angioma possibly induced by an infectious agent. *Glomus tumors* are tender angioneuromas usually located on the fingers and toes.

Angiokeratoma of Mibelli presents dark red to grayish-brown small vascular papules associated with verrucous hyperkeratotic changes of the overlying epidermis. This rare dominant disorder occurs mostly in young persons, predominantly on the extensor surfaces of the fingers and toes and on the knees.

Angiokeratoma of Fordyce occurs as multiple soft red harmless vascular lesions on the scrotum.

Angiokeratoma corporis diffusum of Fabry is a rare, often fatal, familial phospholipid storage disease of smooth muscles of the skin, blood vessels, heart, and kidneys with numerous small angiomatous lesions particularly on the lower trunk of male patients.

Malignant Tumors

Malignant epithelial tumors of the skin generally occur after the fourth decade of life. They may develop in normal or diseased skin. Disorders that sometimes precede cutaneous neoplasms are leukoplakia, xeroderma pigmentosum, senile keratosis or other chronic actinic changes, radiodermatitis, burns, changes due to chronic ingestion of arsenic or prolonged contact with tar products, lupus vulgaris, chronic ulcers, etc. The term *precancerosis* should be used with caution since many "precancerous" lesions show early, superficial cancer (carcinoma in situ) histologically.

Bowen's disease

The usual site of this chronic, slowly progressive squamous cell epithelioma in situ is the skin of the trunk. The individual lesions may range from sharply outlined, maculopapular, round or ovoid patches to polycyclic or vegetating forms with central atrophy. Association with internal cancers is not rare.

Erythroplasia of Queyrat

Circumscribed erythematous velvety patches occur on the glans penis, the prepuce, the vulva, or the oral mucosa. This disorder is related to Bowen's disease.

Paget's disease

Because of its grave prognosis, this disease should never be considered a precancerosis. It represents an intraepidermal carcinoma even in its initial stage. Inconspicuous abnormalities of the female nipple or areola, frequently treated as "eczema" for long periods of time, often represent cancerous changes originating from a mammary duct carcinoma. The prognosis is the same as that of mammary carcinoma. Extramammary lesions may occur in the anogenital region.

Basal cell epithelioma (Basal cell carcinoma)

These tumors are localized most frequently in the upper two-thirds of the face, but may also occur on the trunk (usually as multiple lesions). Their rate of growth is extremely slow. Morphologically, the cellular constituents of these neoplasms resemble basal cells. Metastatic dissemination is virtually absent, but local destruction may be considerable.

Clinical variants are the *nodulo-ulcerative* type (including rodent ulcer), the *cystic* and the *superficial* type, *morphea-like* (fibrosing), *cicatrizing* and *pigmented* basal cell epitheliomas, and the locally invasive *ulcus terebrans* type with deep ulcers and bone involvement.

Squamous cell carcinoma
(Epidermoid carcinoma, Prickle cell cancer)

This tumor combines the usual characteristics of malignancy (destructive, infiltrating growth, metastatic dissemination, general anemia, and cachexia) with a tendency to keratinization or marked dedifferentiation of its cellular elements.

These tumors have a predilection for the mucocutaneous junctions and the mucous membranes. In general, squamous cell carcinomas develop on the basis of chronically inflamed or degenerating cutaneous tissue, rather than in normal skin. Metastatic dissemination to regional lymph nodes and, at an advanced stage, to internal organs may occur. Prognosis differs for specific types of squamous cell carcinoma, such as *carcinoma of the lip, tongue,* and *external genitalia (penis* and *vulva).*

Secondary metastatic tumors of the skin

Malignancies of internal organs rarely metastasize to the skin, whether by hematogenous or lymphogenous dissemination, or by contiguity. The histological structure of such metastatic growths usually reveals the site and structure of the primary tumor. Skin metastases arise most frequently from mammary carcinoma, where lymphogenous dissemination (*lymphangiosis carcinomatosa, carcinoma erysipelatoides*) and/or dissemination by contiguity (*cancer en cuirasse*) may lead to extensive involvement.

Other rare skin metastases arise from malignant melanomas, adenocarcinomas of the gastrointestinal tract, bronchogenic carcinomas, and hypernephromas.

Lentigo maligna
(Melanotic freckle of Hutchinson; Melanosis circumscripta praecancerosa Dubreuilh)

The preferred area of this irregularly pigmented, initially light brown, later almost black macular lesion is the upper portion of the face, but it may occur on any other part of the integument or even on the mucous membranes. Malignant lentigo usually occurs during the latter half of life. In a high percentage of cases, it may develop into a malignant melanoma. Indurated or ulcerating nodules arising from the pigmented lesion are highly suggestive for malignant degeneration.

Malignant melanoma (Melanocarcinoma)

This tumor may occur at any age, but is rare before puberty and reaches its highest incidence in the sixth decade of life.

Malignant melanoma may develop on the basis of degenerating pigmented nevi or malignant lentigo, or may arise from apparently normal skin. The clinical course of this most malignant of human tumors is unpredictable. Differential diagnosis includes all types of pigmented nevi, seborrheic keratoses, granuloma pyogenicum, and Bowen's disease. Melanomas may present as circular, kidney-shaped, or polycyclic lesions. Pigmentation may vary from brown to black. The surface of the lesion is often irregular, sometimes dome-shaped and glistening. Characteristic features are considerable fragility and tendency to hemorrhage. Pinhead-sized satellite tumors are often seen surrounding the primary lesion. There is an extremely great tendency to hematogenous dissemination, even at a relatively early stage. Thus, inconspicuous melanomas of the skin may have metastasized to internal organs before regional lymphadenopathy is demonstrable.

Classification of melanomas according to stages is, therefore, a controversial issue; so are therapeutic suggestions based on such classifications. In the presence of metastases (especially liver metastases) melanoma may be demonstrated by the method of Thormälen and Jaksch. This method is nonspecific; certain drugs may produce false positive reactions.

Sarcomas of the skin

Sarcomas are malignant tumors of mesenchymal origin. They show infiltrating, destructive, and metastatic growth, but do not occur systemically.

Primary sarcomas of the skin originate in the integument and may occur as solitary or multiple tumors. Secondary cutaneous sarcomas spread to the integument as metastases from sarcomas of internal organs or from primary skin sarcomas. The cellular elements of sarcomas resemble embryonic round or spindle cells, reticulum cells, or more highly differentiated mesenchymal tissues (e.g., fibroplastic and angioplastic sarcomas).

Dermatofibrosarcoma protuberans

This mesenchymal tumor develops slowly over a period of several years. The bluish-red, keloid-like, firm, walnut- to fist-sized tumors are frequently found on the chest and in the abdominal region. There is no tendency to necrotic degeneration. Metastatic dissemina-

tion is very rare, but local recurrences are frequent.

Histologically and clinically, this type of tumor assumes an intermediate position between dermatofibroma and fibrosarcoma.

Multiple idiopathic hemorrhagic sarcoma (Kaposi)

Primary lesions often appear in symmetrical distribution on the legs and feet, but may be seen on other parts of the integument. Pinhead- to walnut-sized, dome-shaped, purplish or brownish tumors on legs and feet, often arising from a firm edematous plaque, are the characteristic features of this disease. The angiosarcomatous tumor spreads slowly and may eventually metastasize. Autochthonous new lesions in other areas occur more often than direct metastases from true sarcomatous neoplasms.

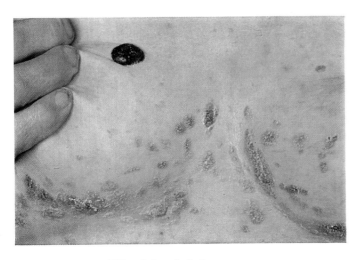

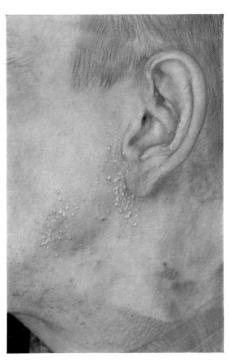

730 Seborrheic keratoses

Numerous sharply circumscribed, raised, soft, yellowish-brown, "stuck-on" tumors with irregular, greasy, scaling surface.

731 Milia

Multiple, round, whitish lesions secondary to trauma.

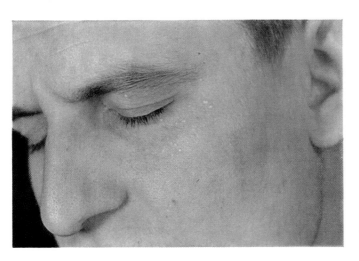

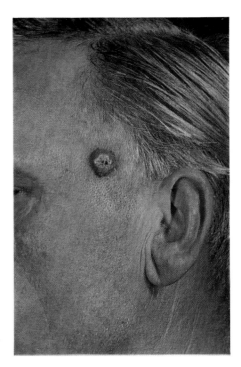

732 Milia. Pinhead-sized, whitish, globoid, firm lesions around the eye, a common localization of spontaneous milia.

733 Keratoacanthoma. Firm, raised, dome-shaped, erythematous tumor with central crater filled with horny masses.

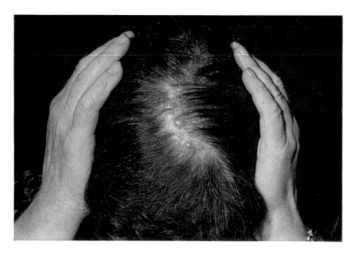

734 Cylindromas (Spiegler tumors)
Multiple, smooth, reddish, round tumors of the scalp with
secondary alopecia.

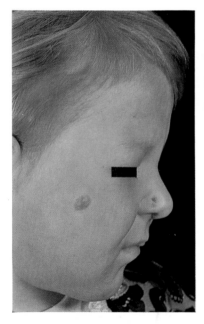

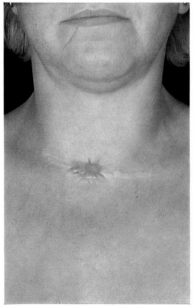

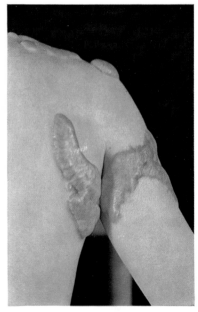

735 Calcifying epithelioma
(MALHERBE)
Solitary, reddish, hard, slightly
raised tumor on the cheek of an
infant.

736 Keloid
Irregular, sharply circumscribed,
raised, red, firm tumor arising
from operation scar.

737 Keloids
Sharply marginated, markedly
raised, hard, red tumors with irregular border and smooth shiny
surface. Secondary to burn.

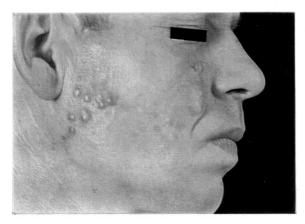

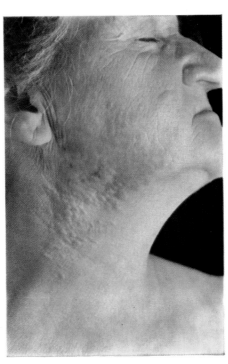

738 Leiomyomas
Multiple, reddish-brown, grouped, firm, painful
nodules of the cheek, sensitive to pressure.

739 Leiomyomas
Large plaque with confluent reddish-
brown firm nodules.

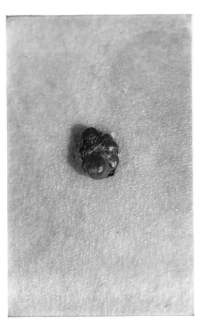

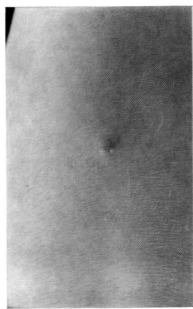

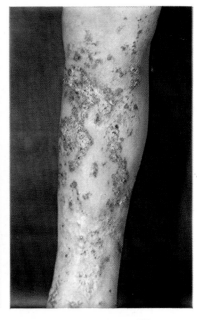

740 Granuloma pyogenicum
Easily bleeding, bright-red, soft,
pedunculated tumor.

741 Glomus tumor
Small, round, deep-seated, bluish-
red, tender nodule on the forearm.

742 Angiokeratoma (MIBELLI)
Grayish-brown, coalescent, vascular papules with marked hyperkeratosis.

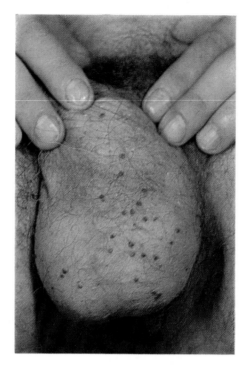

743   Angiokeratoma (FORDYCE)
Multiple, pinhead-sized, brownish-red
vascular lesions of scrotal skin.

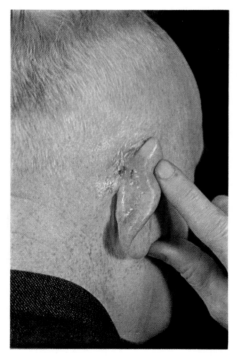

744   Bowen's disease
Sharply marginated erythematous
plaque with smooth glistening surface.

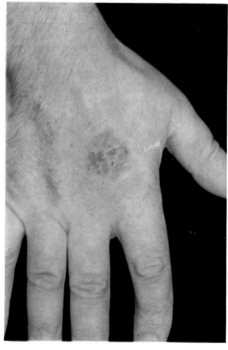

745   Bowen's disease
Circumscribed, round, reddish-brown
patch with irregular scaling surface.

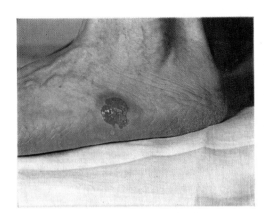

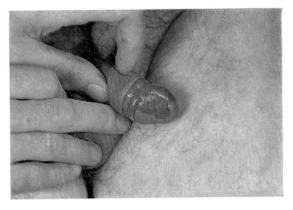

746 Bowen's disease

Sharply outlined, slightly raised, red, eroded plaque on the lateral aspect of the foot.

747 Erythroplasia (Queyrat)

Sharply marginated, red, indolent, nonpruritic, indurated patch with velvety surface and polycyclic border.

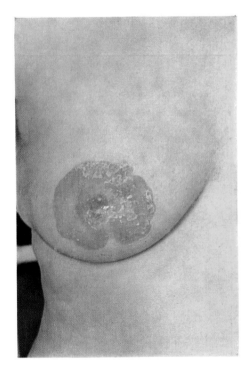

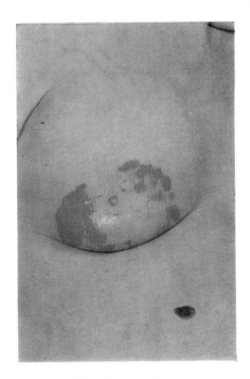

748 Paget's disease

Well defined, oozing, "eczematous," erythematous, scaling changes of the areola (mammary duct carcinoma).

749 Paget's disease

Smooth, red, coalescent plaques of the periareolar area (mammary duct carcinoma).

16*

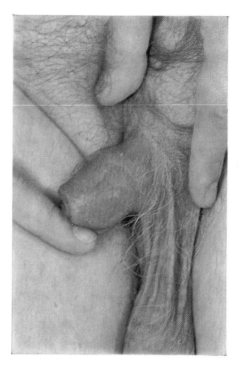

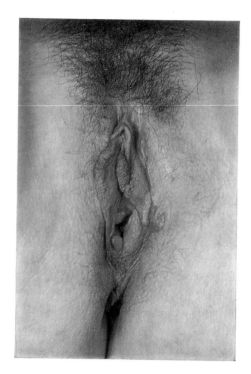

750   Paget's disease

Circumscribed, pink, infiltrated lesion of the penis.

751   Paget's disease

Round, red, slightly raised patch of perivulvar area with smooth surface.

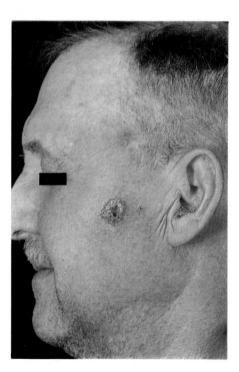

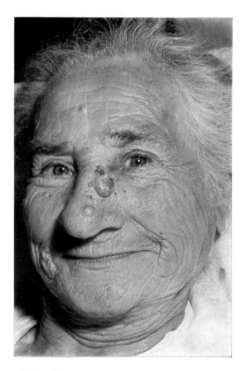

752   Basal cell epithelioma, nodulo-ulcerative type

Firm, round, reddish, scaling nodule with pearly rolled border, central ulceration, and peripheral telangiectases.

753   Basal cell epithelioma, nodulo-ulcerative type

Large, firm, globular tumor with rolled smooth waxy edge and crusted central ulcer.

245

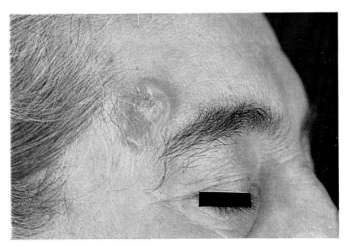

754 **Basal cell epithelioma, nodulo-ulcerative type.** Large, oval, indolent erythematous tumor with smooth, raised, rolled, waxy, nodular border and depressed ulcerated center.

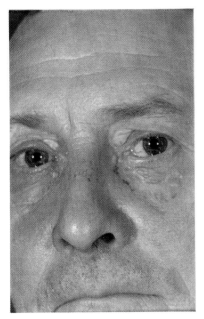

755

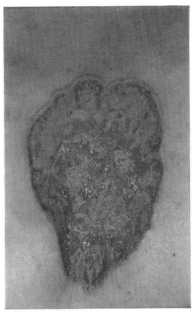

756

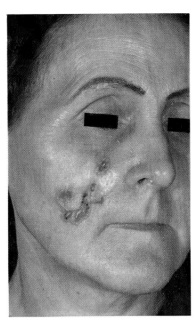

757

755 Basal cell epithelioma, cicatrizing type Of the left lower lid.

756 Basal cell epithelioma, superficial type. Sharply marginated, slightly infiltrated, erythematous, scaling, partially eroded plaque with fine, raised, thread-like, pearly border.

757 Basal cell epithelioma (rodent ulcer) Slowly growing ulcerative and scarring lesion of 20 years duration.

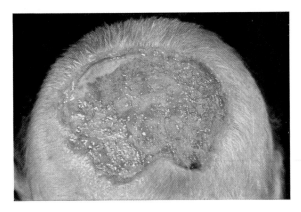

758 Basal cell epithelioma (rodent ulcer). Large, relatively superficial ulcer with granulomatous surface and sharply defined, indurated, nodular pearly border.

246

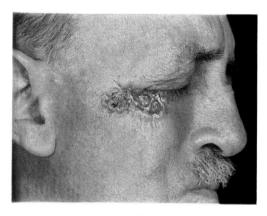

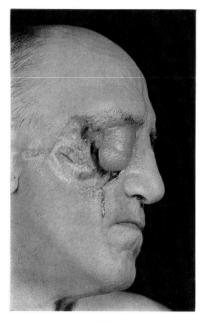

759   **760**

759 and **760**   **Basal cell epithelioma (ulcus terebrans)**
Locally invasive, ulcerative lesion with bone destruction.
Photographs taken three years apart.

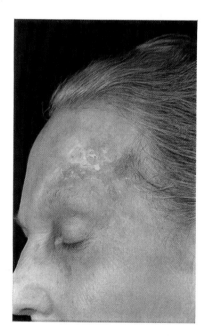

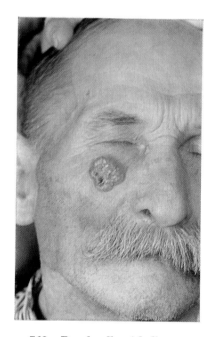

**761   Basal cell epithelioma,
morphea-like type**
On the left side of the forehead
(a common location).

**762   Basal cell epithelioma,
cystic type**
Large, globular, cystic and ulcerating tumor with rolled pearly
border.

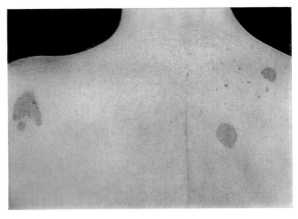

763

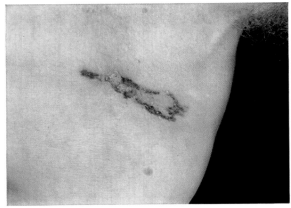

764

763 Basal cell epithelioma, superficial type

Multiple superficial lesions with erythematous, scaling centers and sharply defined, slightly raised, pearly borders.

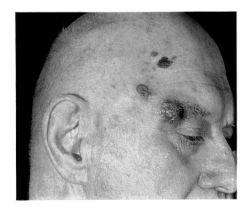

764 Basal cell epithelioma, pigmented type

Ulcerative lesion with nodular, raised, pigmented border.

765 Squamous cell carcinoma

Bright red round tumor with irregular surface and hemorrhagic crust.

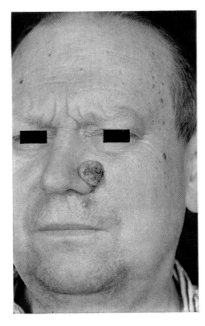

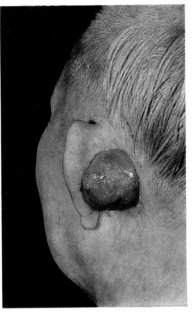

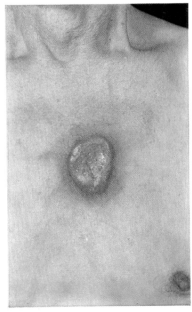

766 Squamous cell carcinoma
Rapidly growing, red, round, elevated, firm, ulcerated tumor.

767 Squamous cell carcinoma
With bowenoid histological features.

768 Squamous cell carcinoma
Bluish-red, rapidly growing, circumscribed, raised tumor with central ulceration.

248

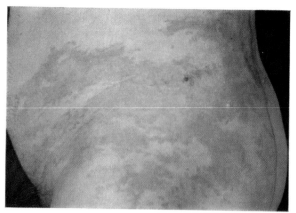

769   Squamous cell carcinoma (carcinoma erysipelatoides)
Cutaneous metastases of squamous cell carcinoma.

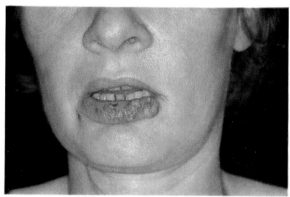

770   Squamous cell carcinoma
Large, infiltrative, firm tumor with nodular
crusted surface on the lower lip.

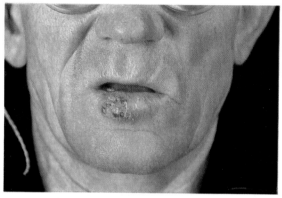

771   Squamous cell carcinoma
Infiltrating firm tumor of the lower lip with irregular scaling and crusted surface.

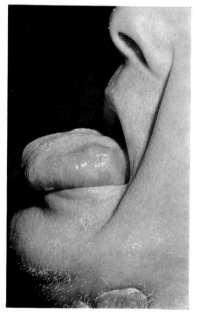

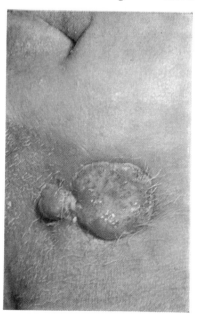

772   **773**

772 and 773   Squamous cell carcinoma
Carcinoma of the tongue, originating from syphilitic glossitis with specific leukoplakia.
Close-up of submandibular metastatic tumor.

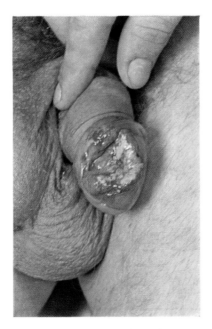

774   Squamous cell carcinoma
Large, destructive, ulcerative tumor of the glans penis.

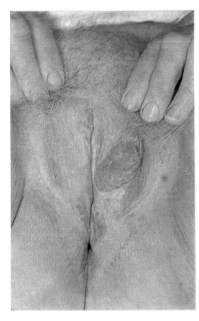

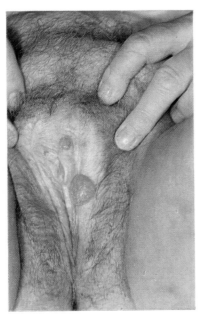

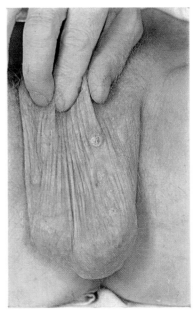

775   Squamous cell carcinoma
Large tumor of the left vulva.

776   Squamous cell carcinoma
Multiple lesions of the vulva.

777   Squamous cell carcinoma
Multiple, small, round tumors of scrotal skin.

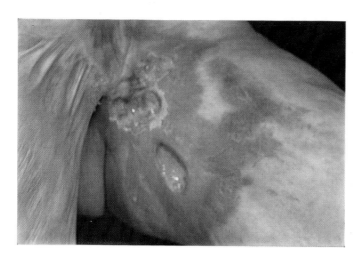

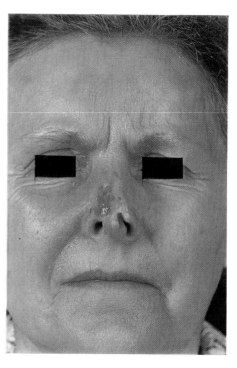

778 Squamous cell carcinoma

Deep, necrotic, destructive ulcers of the thigh originating in scar tissue caused by a burn.

779 Squamous cell carcinoma

Superimposed on lupus vulgaris (carcinoma in lupo).

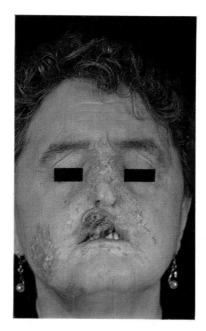

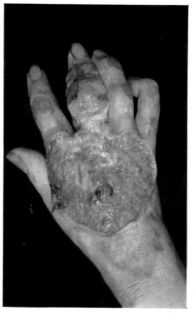

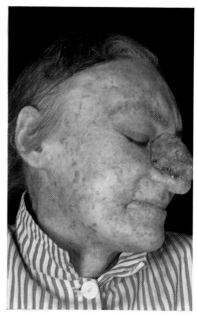

780 Squamous cell carcinoma

Secondary to widespread lupus vulgaris.

781 Squamous cell carcinoma

Extensive ulcerative tumor superimposed on lupus vulgaris lesion.

782 Squamous cell carcinoma

Secondary to extensive chronic discoid lupus erythematosus.

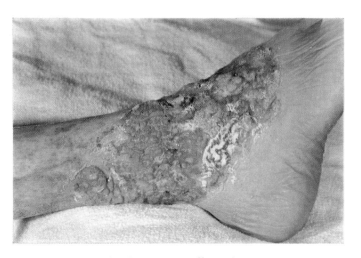

783   Squamous cell carcinoma

Rare complication of acrodermatitis chronica atrophicans HERXHEIMER

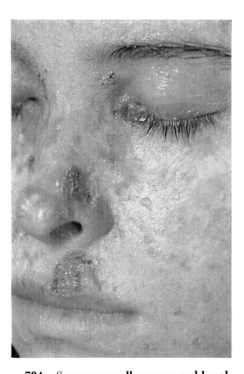

784   Squamous cell cancers and basal cell epitheliomas

In a patient with xeroderma pigmentosum (upper lip, nose, and left lower lid).

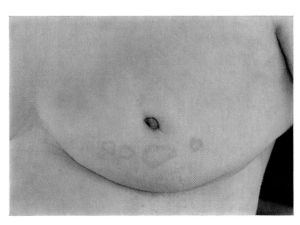

785   Mammary carcinoma

With multiple, erythematous, scaling cutaneous metastases.

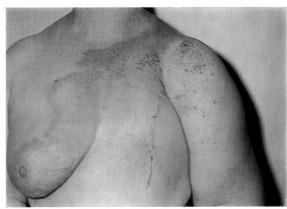

786   Mammary carcinoma

Extensive coalescent, papular and lenticular cutaneous metastases, despite mastectomy and x-ray treatment.

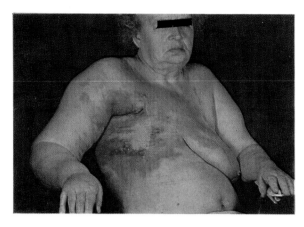

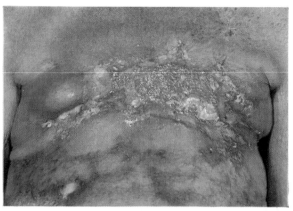

787   Mammary carcinoma
Carcinomatous lymphangiosis resembling erysipelas following mastectomy (carcinoma erysipelatoides).

788   Mammary carcinoma
Diffuse infiltration of the trunk with carcinomatous tissue (cancer en cuirasse).

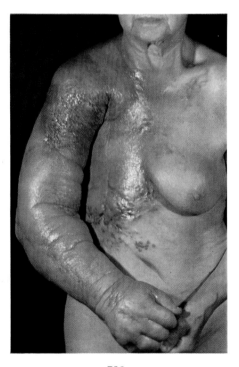

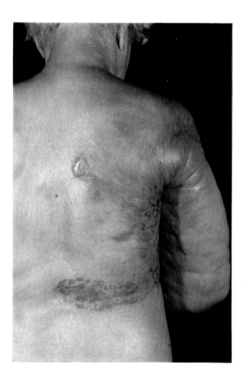

789

790

789 and 790   Mammary carcinoma
Widespread cutaneous metastases with marked lymphedema of the arm, followed by zoster of
T 10 and T 11.

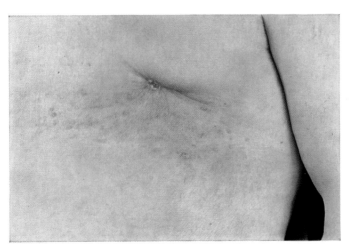

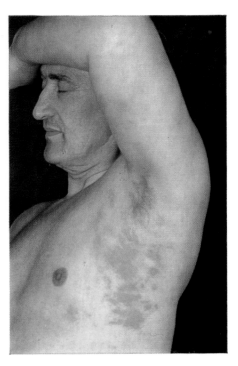

791 Mammary adenocarcinoma
With cutaneous metastases in a male patient.

792 Cutaneous metastases
Of gastric carcinoma.

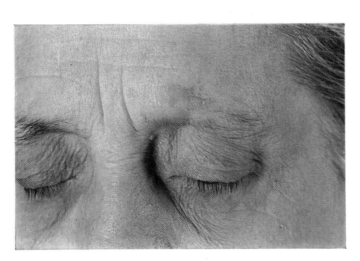

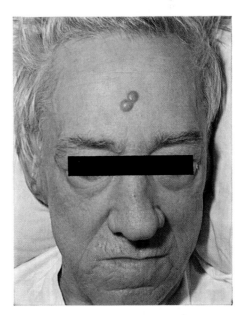

793 Cutaneous metastases
Of an epithelial cancer into the left eyebrow region.

794 Cutaneous metastases
Of bronchogenic carcinoma into the forehead.

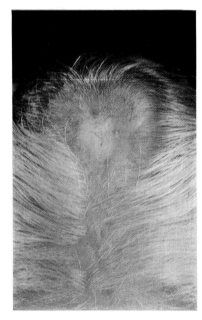

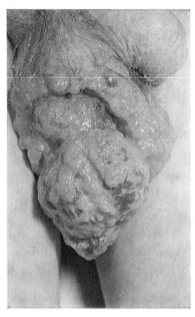

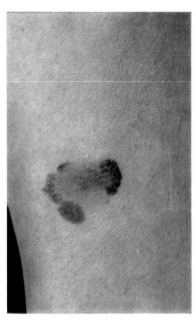

795 Cutaneous metastases

Of adenocarcinoma into the scalp. Primary tumor in gastrointestinal tract.

796 Seminoma

Rare case with widespread involvement of the testes and scrotal skin.

797 Lentigo maligna (Hutchinson's freckle)

Sharply circumscribed macular hyperpigmentation.

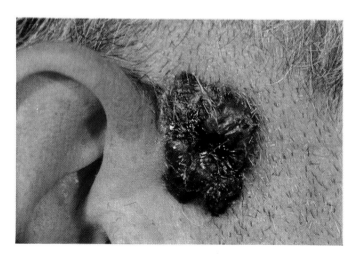

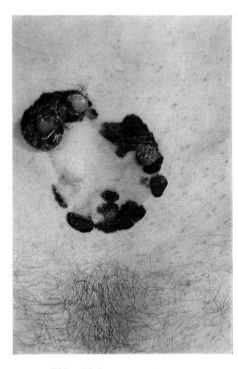

798 Malignant melanoma

Large, raised, hemorrhagic, black tumor derived from lentigo maligna.

799 Malignant melanoma

Nodular lesions developing in preexisting macular lentigo maligna.

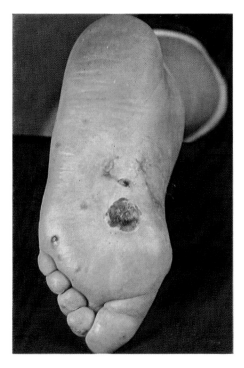

800   Malignant melanoma
Ulcerated, granulomatous, pigmented
lesion of the foot.

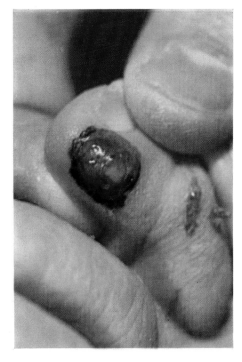

801   Malignant melanoma
Raised granulomatous tumor of the toe
with sharply marginated black border.

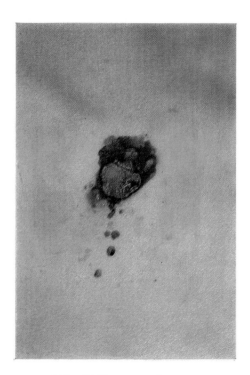

802   Malignant melanoma
With local metastases due to lymphogenous dissemination.

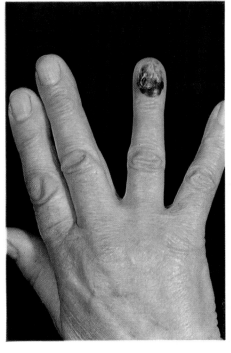

803   Malignant melanoma
Of subungual and periungual region
(melanotic whitlow).

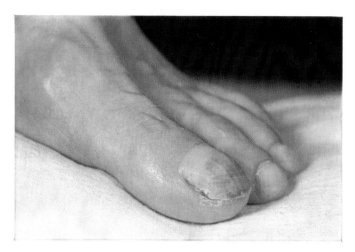

804   Malignant melanoma

Subungual lesion originating from the nail bed.

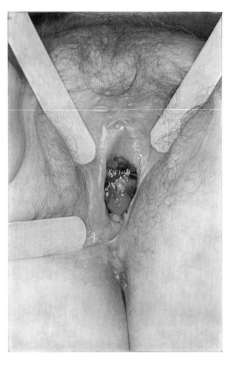

805   Malignant melanoma

Of mucous membrane of the vagina.

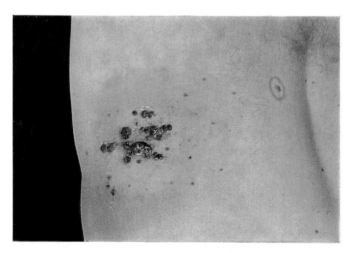

806   Malignant melanoma

Small, paravertebral primary tumor with multiple lymphogenous metastases into the skin of the lateral aspect of the abdomen.

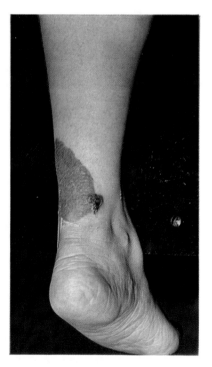

807   Malignant melanoma

Arising from the border of a pigmented nevus of long duration.

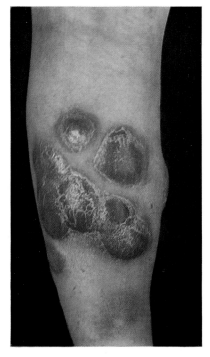

808 Reticulum cell sarcoma

Indolent, purplish nodes of the lower leg with a tendency to ulcerative degeneration.

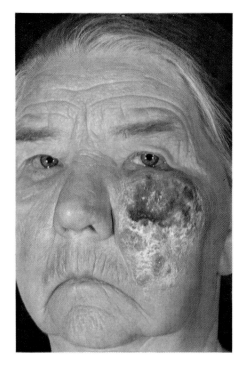

809 Reticulum cell sarcoma

Large, firm, irregular, ulcerated tumor of the left cheek.

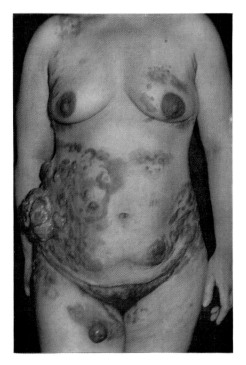

810 Reticulosarcomatosis (GOTTRON)

Multicentric development during pregnancy; no primary tumor.

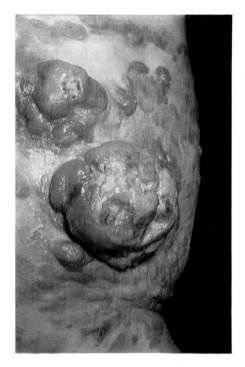

811 Reticulosarcomatosis (GOTTRON)

Close-up view of the large tumors shown in figure 810.

258

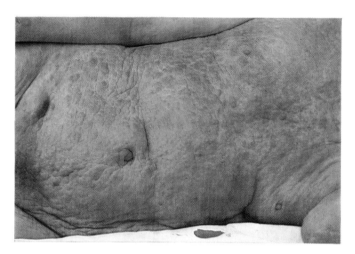

812   Reticulosarcomatosis (GOTTRON)

Widespread lesions on the chest and abdomen resembling
a nonspecific maculopapular eruption.

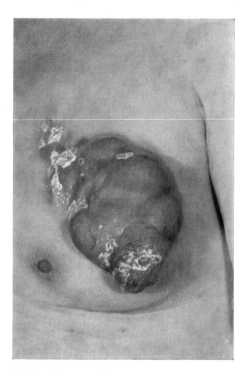

813   Dermatofibrosarcoma protuberans

Large, firm, indolent, bluish-red tumor
with irregular surface on the upper chest.

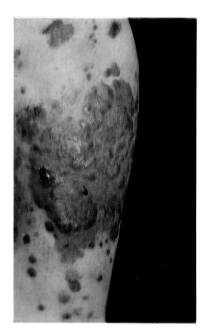

**814   Multiple idiopathic
hemorrhagic sarcoma** (KAPOSI)

Coalescent and isolated, firm, angiomatous tumors of the lower leg.

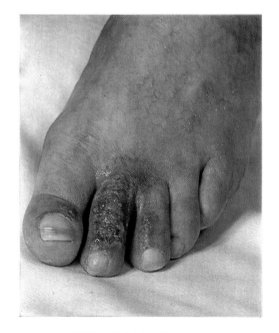

**815   Multiple idiopathic
hemorrhagic sarcoma** (KAPOSI)

Irritated exudative lesions of the toes with
firm edema of the dorsum of the foot.

Venereal Diseases and Diseases of the External Genitals

The term venereal diseases is commonly applied to infections transmitted by sexual contact, such as syphilis, chancroid, lymphogranuloma venereum, and gonorrhea. In rare cases, these diseases may be acquired without direct contact. Other disorders involving the external genitals, such as balanoposthitis in men and ulcus vulvae acutum in women, develop independently of sexual intercourse. Finally, certain cutaneous and infectious disorders predominantly affecting other areas of the body may be localized occasionally on the genital organs.

Syphilis

Syphilis is a chronic infectious disease, as are tuberculosis and leprosy. The causative organism, Treponema pallidum, is a slender spiral consisting of 6 to 20 (usually 8 to 12) tightly arranged coils. The organism is actively motile, rotating around its long axis.

Treponema pallidum (Spirochaeta pallida) was discovered by SCHAUDINN in cooperation with HOFFMANN (1905). Because of its poor stainability, the parasite was named "Spirochaeta pallida." It enters the human organism through damaged skin or mucous membranes, unless it is introduced directly into the blood stream, as by blood transfusions. Infection may be genital, perigenital, or extragenital. The most common form of direct transmission is by sexual contact; indirect transmission may occur through jointly used spoons, glasses, lipsticks, cigarettes, etc.

Primary syphilis

The typical cutaneous manifestation of the primary state of early syphilis is the *chancre* (rarely in the form of multiple chancres). It appears 3 to 4 weeks after infection in the anogenital region or at any other site where the treponemes have entered the body. Usually, it is a flat, round or oblong, indurated maculopapular lesion of varying size. The overlying skin generally macerates and develops into a smooth, clean erosion, which exudes a serous fluid. Untreated primary lesions may develop superficial erosions and finally form an indurated ulcer (ulcus durum), especially when located on the lips, the glans, the coronal fold, or the tonsils. A single, nontender, firm, enlarged regional lymph node occurs shortly after appearance of the chancre.

Treponemes obtained from exudate of primary lesions may best be demonstrated by *darkfield microscopy;* they are visualized as light, colorless spirals. In special cases various stains, silver techniques, and india ink preparations may be used. The darkfield technique, however, is the quickest, simplest, and most reliable method. Darkfield examination of oral lesions is difficult because of the presence of other normally occuring treponemes.

Secondary syphilis

The secondary stage of early syphilis is reached 7 to 10 weeks after infection (seldom later), and is usually preceded by prodromal symptoms such as headaches, malaise, backaches, and slightly elevated temperature. (Rarely, secondary syphilitic eruptions may occur several years after infection, sometimes as recurrent episodes.) The lesions consist of superficial, circumscribed tissue reactions induced by predominantly perivascular accumulations of treponemes. Involvement of other organs may be overt (general lymphadenopathy, pharyngitis, nephritis, periostitis, iritis, myositis, "motheaten" patchy alopecia, meningovascular reactions with changes in cerebrospinal fluid) or latent. Serological tests are positive in 100 per cent of patients in this stage. They first become positive within 2 to 3 weeks after the appearance of the primary lesion.

In spite of their great variability, secondary syphilitic skin lesions (secondary syphilids) show certain clinical characteristics which separate them from similar eruptions. They prefer the trunk in symmetrical distribution (syphilitic roseola); the face (except in Negroes) and extensor surfaces of the extremities are less frequently involved. Macular lesions of palms and soles are fairly common. Secondary lesions appear suddenly within 4 to 5 days; marked inflammatory changes are absent. Fresh macular lesions show a bright red, older ones a darker (raw ham) color. Tenderness, pruritus, vesiculation, and scaling are lacking; there is no marked elevation of body temperature. The lesions contain numerous treponemes. When the overlying skin is eroded, the lesions are highly contagious. They subside without leaving marks or scars. In exceptional cases, older regressing papular exanthemas may be scaly, micropapular exanthemas may be pruritic, or pustular eruptions may leave small scars. Annular lesions, often showing bizarre configuration and central hyperpigmentation, are more common in Negroes.

The *initial macular or papular exanthema* of the secondary stage of syphilis represents the most conspicuous eruption, whereas the second and third *recurrent exanthemas*, which occasionally follow, show fewer but larger lesions; their tendency to grouping increases with time, thus marking the transition to the late (tertiary) stage.

Latent syphilis

The latent stage of syphilis is characterized by complete absence of symptoms except reactive serologic tests. Since the disease is continuous, no sharp line can be drawn between early latent and late latent syphilis. Most authors classify early latent syphilis as syphilis of less than 4 years' duration, and late latent syphilis as syphilis of more than 4 years' duration.

Late syphilis

The classification of late syphilis includes asymptomatic and symptomatic neurosyphilis (paresis, tabes dorsalis, and meningovascular neurosyphilis), cardiovascular syphilis (aortic insufficiency or aortic aneurysm), and late benign syphilis (cutaneous, osseous, and visceral gumma). The most common cutaneous forms of *late benign (tertiary) syphilis* are solitary *gummas* (often with typical punched-out ulcers), and *nodular-ulcerative (tubero-serpiginous) syphilids*, which usually show an arciform, gyrate, polycyclic or annular pattern. These lesions are painless and nonpruritic, as were those of secondary syphilis; otherwise,

they are entirely different from the lesions of early syphilis: their distribution is asymmetrical and they develop slowly over periods of weeks or months, always leaving atrophic or cicatricial changes. They contain few treponemes and are virtually noncontagious. The same is true of late mucosal lesions and changes of internal organs.

The site of secondary and late syphilitic lesions of the skin and mucous membranes is often determined by chronic irritation. During the secondary stage, physiologic and pathologic excretions often induce condylomata lata in the vicinity of body orifices. Late skin manifestations of the tertiary stage occasionally occur at the site of morphine, bismuth, or mercury injections given in the past, near injuries caused by shell fragments, after repeated x-irradiation or other forms of chronic irritation.

The term *syphilis d'emblée* is applied to manifestations of the secondary stage not preceded by primary lesions, as in transfusion syphilis, congenital syphilis, or after insufficient prophylactic treatment.

However, not all cases of syphilis that appear to start with the secondary stage are cases of syphilis d'emblée; especially in women, the primary lesions may have been overlooked because of their obscure localization (vagina, cervix).

An unusual type of acquired syphilis in its early stage is *syphilis maligna*, which is characterized by ulcerative mucocutaneous lesions, severe constitutional symptoms, frequently negative serologic tests for syphilis, and absence of generalized lymphadenopathy.

Clinical diagnosis of syphilitic lesions is supported by darkfield studies and nontreponemal antigen reactions (serologic test for syphilis = STS), particulary precipitation and complement fixation tests. More specific results can be obtained with treponemal antigen tests, especially the Treponema Pallidum Immobilization (TPI) test (NELSON) and fluorescent treponemal antibody tests.

Biologic false positive (BFP) serologic reactions may occur after smallpox vaccination, in malaria, infectious mononucleosis, systemic lupus erythematosus, rheumatoid arthritis and other systemic diseases.

Acquired syphilis takes a predictable course up to the beginning of the secondary stage; its later development is variable. Not every patient develops late syphilis. Only in a small percentage of all patients who remained untreated or were treated insufficiently, the skin manifestations of *late syphilis* may occur. The disease may enter a latent period without being cured. Thus a positive serologic test may be found in apparently perfectly healthy persons, e.g., during premarital examination. Others may develop late manifestations without ever having known of their disease or having been treated for it.

Congenital syphilis may be demonstrated in the fetus from the end of the fourth month of pregnancy. It is due exclusively to transmission by the syphilitic mother. There is no true primary lesion. The infection proceeds gradually via the placenta and spreads through the entire fetal organism. Therefore, the course of this disease is different from that of postnatally acquired syphilis. Changes in internal organs take place before birth and remain noticeable postnatally. At birth, secondary lesions (roseola, papules) may be present. For periods of many years, the same eruptions as in acquired syphilis may occur, although spaced more irregularly. Not infrequently, infants with congenital syphilis are dehydrated and marasmic; the most common congenital symptoms are bullous lesions on palms and soles, syphilitic pemphigoid, rhinitis ("snuffles"), and rhagades of the perioral region. Characteristic late *stigmata* of congenital syphilis persisting throughout life are radial perioral rhagades, frontal or parietal bosses, sabre shins, high palatine arch, saddle nose, Hutchinsonian teeth and mulberry molars.

Chancroid
(Ulcus molle)

After an incubation period of 1 to 3 days, small, usually multiple, inflammatory erythematous tender macules, vesicles, or pustules appear; they rupture early to form soft purulent ulcers with ragged undermined borders. Smears taken from the edges often show Hemophilus ducreyi (Streptobacillus DUCREY-UNNA), a gram-negative rod, in typical "school of fish" arrangement. The genital lesion of chancroid, transmitted almost exclusively by sexual intercourse, is characterized by a *soft* ulcer. Occasionally, this is raised above the level of the surrounding skin. Less frequently, rapid degeneration — probably due to mixed infection — may occur, producing the clinical picture of gangrenous chancroid. Involvement of regional lymph nodes is frequently seen in

the form of a unilateral bubo, which is tender (in contrast to syphilis) and may ulcerate spontaneously.

An important complication is simultaneous infection with syphilis. Repeated serologic tests for syphilis are imperative. The diagnosis of chancroid is confirmed by demonstration of the microorganisms, autoinoculation (inoculation in abdominal skin), and a skin test with Ducrey vaccine (ITO-REENSTIERNA test) which becomes positive after the appearance of bubos.

Lymphogranuloma venereum
(Lymphogranuloma inguinale)
(DURAND-NICOLAS-FAVRE)

Following an incubation period of 2 to 6 weeks, an inconspicuous evanescent vesicular or ulcerating primary lesion appears, usually on the external genitals. Two to four weeks later, male patients (predominantly Negroes) develop unilateral (less frequently bilateral) inguinal lymphadenitis. Characteristically, the nodes in a chain fuse together in a large mass. Occasionally, the bubos break down and form fistulous openings. From the inguinal area, the process spreads to the intra-abdominal lymph nodes. In female patients having a primary lesion on the cervix, the process directly affects the pelvic lymph nodes. The microorganism causing lymphogranuloma venereum is a virus related to the rickettsiae, which was discovered by MIYAGAWA in 1935. Diagnostic aids are the complement fixation test and the intradermal FREI test.

Esthiomene (elephantiasis of the female genitals) and strictures or ulcerations of the anorectal region secondary to a primary proctitis represent advanced stages of lymphogranuloma venereum. Cancers of the rectum and adjacent areas have been reported.

Granuloma Inguinale
(Granuloma venereum)
(DONOVAN)

This venereal disease, which occurs predominantly in Negroes, is characterized by sharply circumscribed, indolent, granulating, and vegetating ulcerations on the external genitals and in the groin, usually without lymphadenopathy. The causative organism (Donovania granulomatis) is gram-negative and may be stained with the Giesmsa stain (Donovan bodies).

Gonorrhea

Gonorrhea is still a serious venereal disease; careful diagnosis and adequate therapy are imperative.

Neisseria gonorrhoeae, a gram-negative diplococcus, was discovered by NEISSER in 1879. The organism is easily demonstrated in smears stained with methylene blue. Cultures may be made in special cases (e.g., in the presence of complications of gonorrhea in women, or in order to ascertain that the disease has been cured). While the micrococci may survive and retain their infectiousness for hours in a moist environment (towels, bath sponges, etc.) infection without sexual intercourse is excedingly rare.

After an incubation period of 1 to 8 days, a creamy, yellowish-green, purulent urethral discharge appears. If this acute anterior gonorrheal urethritis is treated inadequately or not at all, it may develop into gonorrheal cavernitis, paraurethral infiltrations, posterior gonorrheal urethritis (and later urethral strictures), gonorrheal prostatitis, involvement of the seminal vesicles, funiculitis, and finally, gonorrheal epididymitis.

In the sexually mature female, the disease may involve the urethra, SKENE's ducts, BARTHOLIN's ducts, and the cervix. The squamous cell epithelium and the acidity of the vagina prevent gonorrheal vaginitis. Possible complications of gonorrhea in female patients are endometritis, salpingitis, oophoritis, and peritonitis. Infantile gonorrheal vulvo-vaginitis presents special therapeutic problems. The vestibulum and vagina of the infant are especially vulnerable to invasion by gonococci. The urethra and cervix usually are also involved. In school-age girls, complications of ascending gonorrhea must be taken into consideration.

Extragenital gonorrheal infections are *gonoblennorrhea neonatorum* and *gonoblennorrhea adultorum* (gonorrheal conjunctivitis).

Yaws
(Frambesia, Pian)

Yaws is not a venereal disease. Unlike syphilis, it is usually transmitted through direct extragenital contact. The causative organism, Treponema pertenue, resembles Treponema pallidum in appearance, motility, and stainability; it was discovered by CASTELLANI in 1905. The close relationship between syphilis and yaws justifies discussion of the latter in this context.

Infection is extragenital in about 99 per cent of all cases; in approximately 90 per cent, this takes place during childhood. The microorganism enters the host organism through small injuries, fissures, or scratches. The primary lesions often appear on the lower extremities. The disease, which is confined to tropical and subtropical regions, starts after an incubation period of 2 to 4 weeks with a small papule or pustule; prodromal symptoms are fairly common. This *primary lesion* rapidly grows, erodes, and forms a crust. Occasionally, papillomatous or ulcerative primary lesions are seen. They subside after 6 weeks, or may persist for several months.

The *secondary stage* is usually preceded by generalized lymphadenopathy. Manifestation of the secondary stage, characterized by an exanthematous eruption, may take from 3 weeks to 3 months; predilection areas are the extremities and the face. The initial exanthema consists of small papules; some regress, but the majority develop into larger papillomas with superficial granulating erosions. It is from this raspberry-like appearance of the lesions (raspberry = framboise) that the disease derives its name. The lesions may coalesce, giving rise to large ulcerations. The secondary stage is characterized by frequent recurrences over periods ranging from several months to two years. A latent period follows which may either terminate the disease or mark the transition to the *tertiary or late stage*. This shows isolated lesions resembling those of tertiary syphilis, which lead to extensive tissue destruction. Severe osseous involvement may occur, resulting in deformities. *Gangosa* (rhinopharyngitis mutilans) is a special form of tertiary yaws; it causes severe mutilations of nose and palate, destroying soft tissue as well as bone and cartilage.

Serological tests for syphilis are positive in yaws.

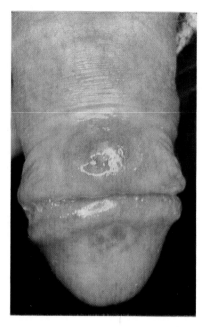

816 Primary syphilis (chancre)

Typical early indurated clean lesion. Numerous treponemes demonstrated by darkfield microscopy. Serologic tests for syphilis (STS) were negative.

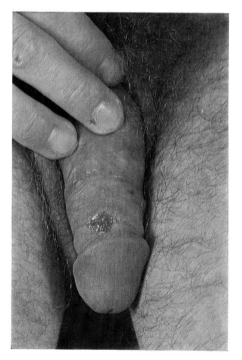

817 Primary syphilis (chancre)

Smooth, clean, exudative, infiltrated, erosive lesion. Darkfield positive; STS negative.

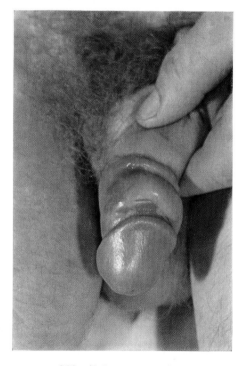

818 Primary syphilis

Multiple, erosive, infiltrated lesions. Darkfield positive; STS negative.

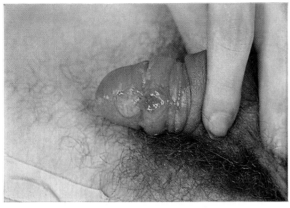

819 Primary syphilis (chancre)
Indolent, indurated, plate-like lesion showing incipient ulceration (ulcus durum). Darkfield positive; STS negative.

821 Primary syphilis (chancre). Indurated ulcer on the shaft of the penis. Darkfield positive; STS negative.

822 Primary syphilis (chancre). Firm clean ulcer on mons pubis (ulcus durum). Darkfield positive.

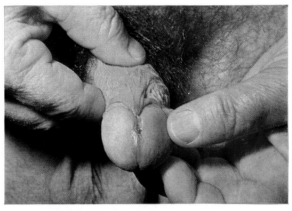

820 Primary syphilis (chancre)
Small, firm, indolent, ulcerative lesion of the frenulum. Darkfield positive.

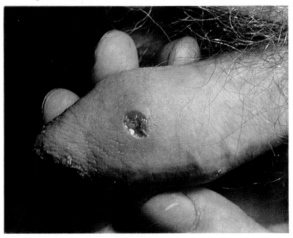

821

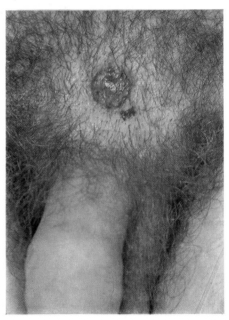

822

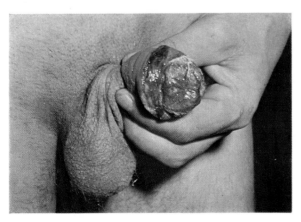

823 Primary syphilis
Marked necrotic degeneration (phagedenic chancre). STS positive.

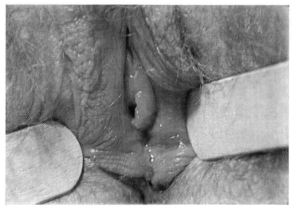

824 Primary syphilis (chancre)
Flat, firm, indolent, ulcerative lesion of fourchette. Darkfield positive; STS negative.

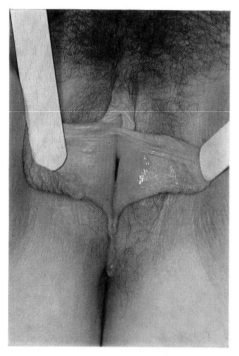

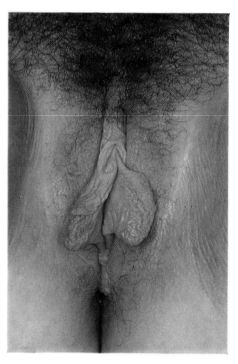

825 Primary syphilis

Multiple, infiltrated, erosive chancres on internal aspect of the labia minora. Darkfield positive; STS negative.

826 Primary syphilis (chancre)

Small, round, indurated ulcer on internal aspect of the right labium minus. Primary lesions of the external female genitals are less common than internal genital lesions.

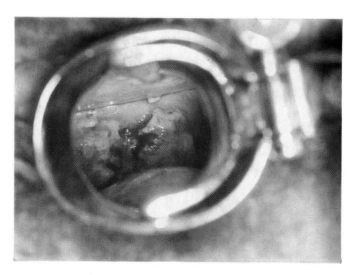

827 Primary syphilis (chancre)

Indurated vaginal ulcer. Such lesions are frequently missed.

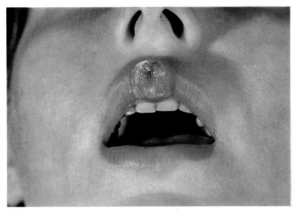

828   Primary syphilis (chancre)

Large indurated lesion on the upper lip.
Darkfield positive; STS positive.

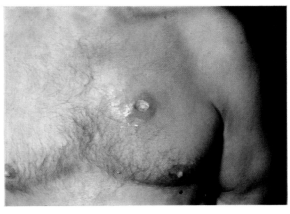

829   Primary syphilis (chancre)

Extragenital lesion on the chest with ulcerative
degeneration. Infection probably due to bite injury.
Darkfield and STS positive.

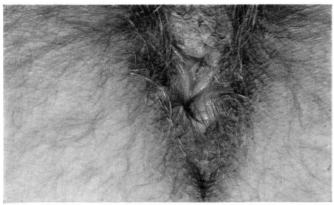

830   Primary syphilis (chancre)

Indurated ulcer of the anal region, easily confused
with fissures. Darkfield positive; STS negative.

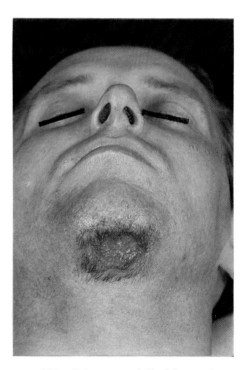

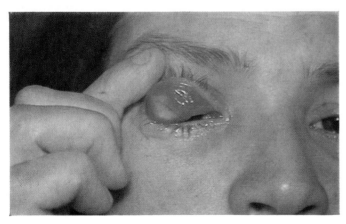

831   Primary syphilis (chancre)

Indolent firm ulcer on internal aspect of the upper eyelid,
with regional lymphadenopathy. Transmission by wiping
eye with handkercief previously used on grandchild suffering
from syphilitic coryza.

832   Primary syphilis (chancre)

Large indurated ulcer of the chin.
Darkfield and STS positive.

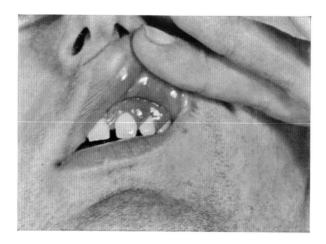

833 Primary syphilis (chancre)
Painless, easily bleeding, rapidly growing ulcer of gums
with regional lymphadenopathy.

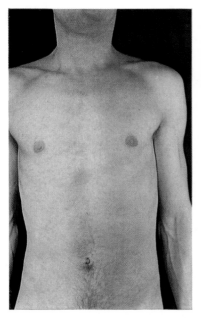 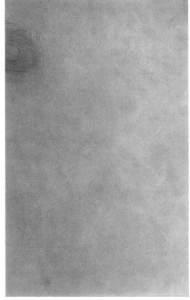 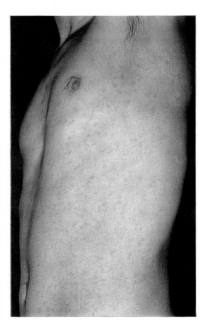

834 Secondary syphilis (syphilitic roseola)	**835 Secondary syphilis (syphilitic roseola)**	**836 Secondary syphilis (syphilitic roseola)**
Evenly distributed, macular ex-anthema consisting mostly of round lesions; macular syphilid.	Close-up view of macular eruption. Darkfield and STS positive.	Macular exanthema with round or oval lesions which follow the lines of cleavage of the skin.

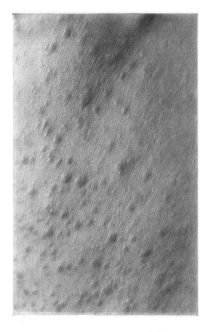

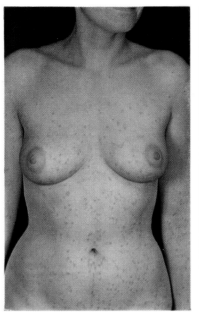

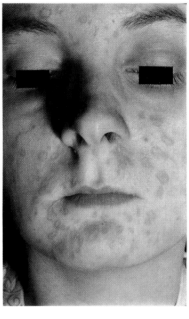

**837   Secondary syphilis
(syphilitic roseola)**

Slightly raised lesions, not as sharply defined as those of the papular exanthematous variety.

838   Secondary syphilis

Papular syphilid with sharply defined, round, raised infiltrations of "raw ham color". Individual papules are tender to pressure with a small probe (Ollendorff sign).

839   Secondary syphilis

Erythematosquamous syphilid of the face, simulating seborrheic dermatitis.

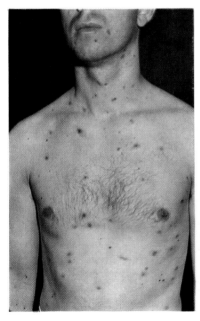

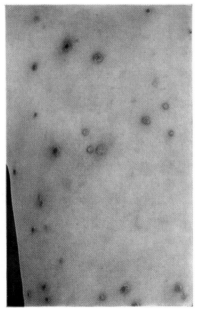

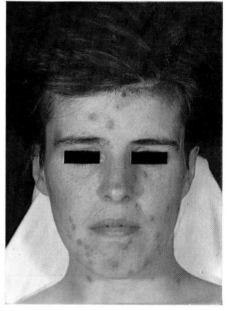

840   Secondary syphilis

Necrotic degeneration of some papules leads to small, crusted ulcerations.

841   Secondary syphilis

Scattered, varicelliform papulo-pustular lesions (recurrent exanthema). A rare variety.

842   Secondary syphilis

Papulosquamous syphilid of the face.

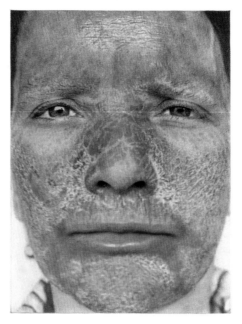

843 Secondary syphilis

Tuberculoid syphilid with brownish-red, soft, scaling lesions
in patchy distribution covering the entire face. Diascopy
reveals infiltrations resembling lupus vulgaris nodules. Rare
manifestation of late secondary syphilis.

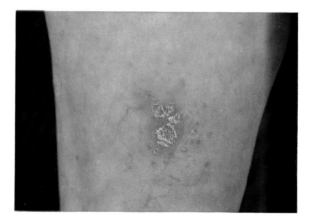

844 Secondary syphilis

Corymbose syphilid with small papules grouped in a circle
around a large central papule in late secondary syphilis.

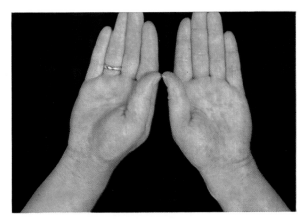

845

845 and **846** **Secondary syphilis**
Reddish-brown, slightly scaling, dry, macular and papular symmetrical lesions of the palms. Involvement of palms and soles, in combination with other symptoms is highly suggestive of secondary syphilis.

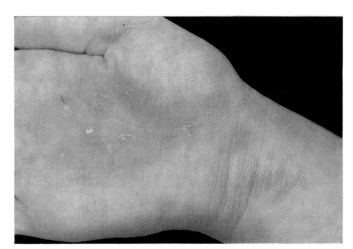

846

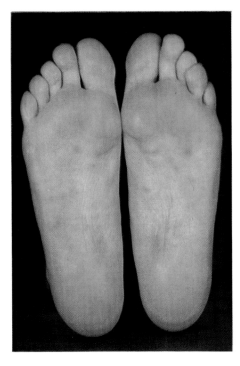

847

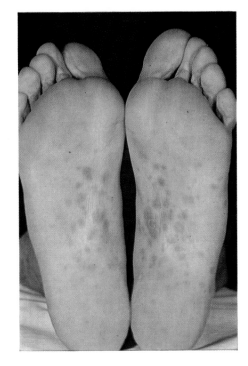

848

847 and **848** **Secondary syphilis.** Round, scaling, maculopapular lesions of the soles.

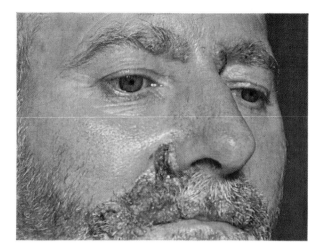

849   Secondary syphilis

Granulating yellow masses on the eyebrows and nasolabial folds in a diabetic patient, resembling yaws. These granulating lesions are rare and usually seen in seborrheic regions.

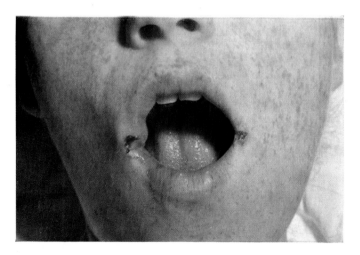

850   Secondary syphilis

"Split papules" of the corners of the mouth, resembling perlèche.

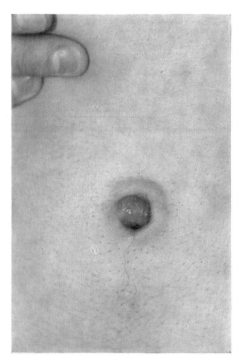

851   Secondary syphilis

Syphilitic papules in the navel. Macerated, oozing lesions may also occur in the interdigital areas.

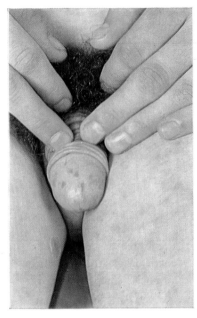

852 Secondary syphilis
Eroded syphilitic papules on the glans penis.

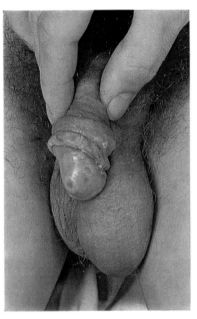

853 Secondary syphilis
Mucous patches on the glans penis and internal lamina of the prepuce.

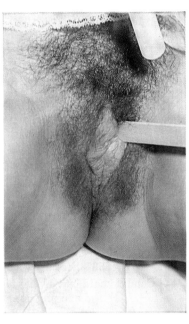

854 Secondary syphilis
Mucous patches on the internal aspect of the labia minora.

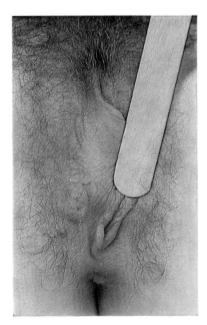

855 Secondary syphilis
Condylomata lata of the labia majora.

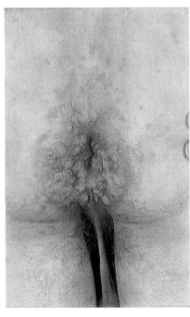

856 Secondary syphilis
Condylomata lata of the anus.

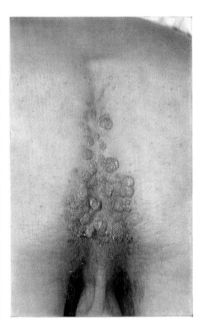

857 Secondary syphilis
Condylomata lata of the anus.

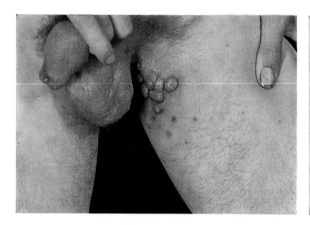

858 Secondary syphilis
Condylomata lata of the thigh, scrotum,
and prepuce.

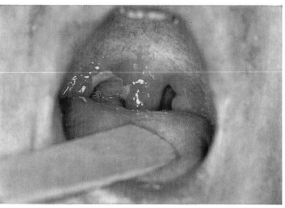

859 Secondary syphilis
Syphilitic tonsillitis with smooth papular
lesions.

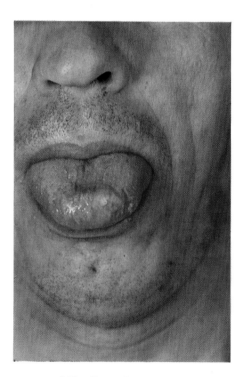

860 Secondary syphilis
Flat, slightly raised syphilitic papules
on the tongue.

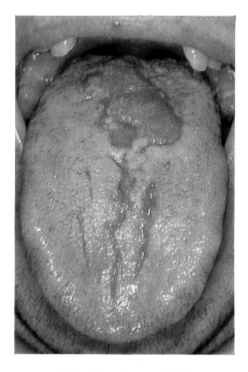

861 Secondary syphilis
Flat, smooth papules on the tip of the
tongue; coalescent, raised lesions on
the dorsum of the tongue.

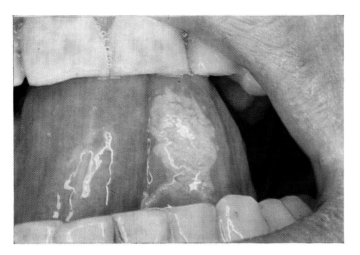

862 Secondary syphilis

Mucous patches of the underside of the tongue.

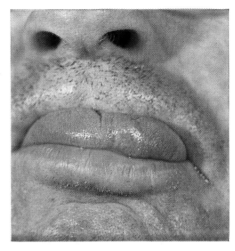

863 Secondary syphilis

Circumscribed, whitish, shallow erosions on the tip of the tongue
(opaline patch).

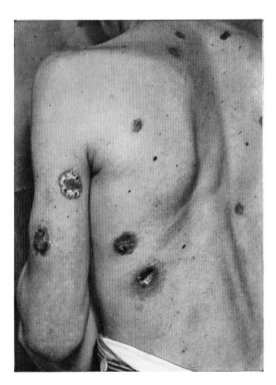

864 Syphilis maligna

Primary ulcerative lesions of the trunk.
STS negative.

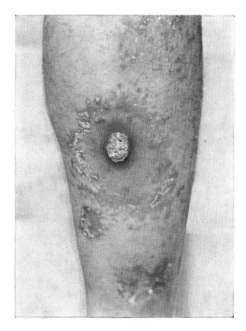

865 Syphilis maligna

Densely grouped and scattered satellite
lesions surrounding a larger central
lesion.

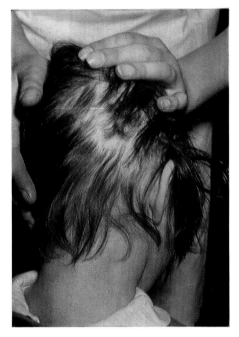

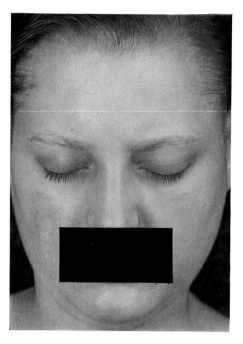

866   Secondary syphilis

Syphilitic alopecia with typical
"moth-eaten" appearance of the scalp
in a 4-year-old girl with acquired
syphilis.

867   Secondary syphilis

Syphilitic alopecia of the eyebrows and
eyelashes in early syphilis.

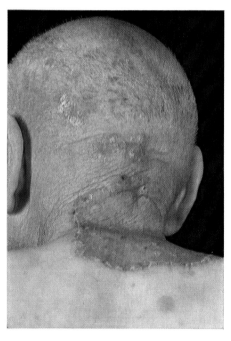

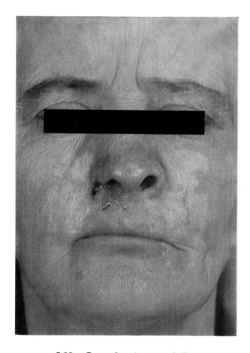

868   Late benign syphilis

Nodulo-ulcerative tertiary syphilis on
the nape and scalp with serpiginous
border. STS positive.

869   Late benign syphilis

Tuberoserpiginous tertiary syphilis.
Ivory-colored scars with erythematous,
inflamed margins represent the healed
portion of the lesion which continues to
spread peripherally.

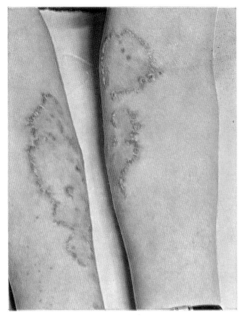

870   Late benign syphilis

Bilateral, symmetrical, nodulo-ulcerative syphilis on the forearms. Usually not found in symmetrical distribution; early manifestations of late syphilis occasionally may depart from that pattern. Serpiginous borders and scarring are characteristic of late syphilis. STS positive.

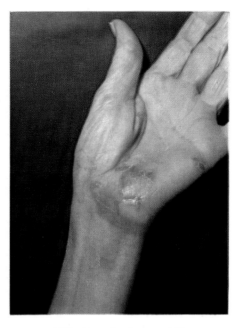

871   Late benign syphilis

Nodulo-ulcerative syphilis, with concomitant inconspicuous scars on the trunk. STS positive.

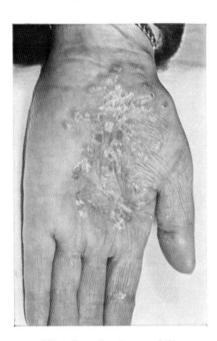

872   Late benign syphilis

Nodulo-ulcerative syphilis of the palm. Manifestations of late syphilis on the palms and soles frequently lose the characteristic features that they present elsewhere. Absence of pruritus and pain, unilateral occurrence, and positive STS help differentiate this eruption.

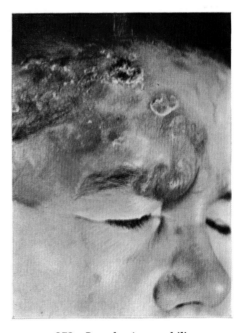

873   Late benign syphilis

Cicatrizing tuberoserpiginous syphilis on the temples. The borders indicate that the tumor developed from firm, densely grouped papular lesions. STS positive.

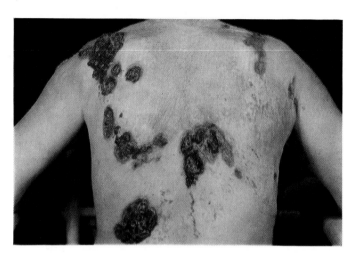

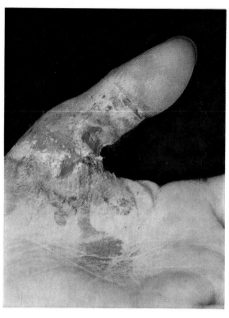

874   Late benign syphilis

Ulcerated, grouped, tuberoserpiginous syphilis which has spread over large areas of the back, as shown by the residual hyperpigmented scars.

875   Late benign syphilis

Deep punched-out gummatous ulcer of the thumb.

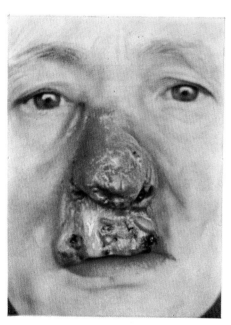

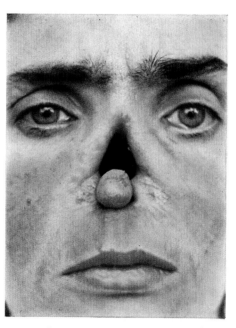

876   Late benign syphilis

Gummatous lesion on the upper lip and nose.

877   Late benign syphilis

Destruction of the osseous and cartilaginous structures of the nose (gumma).

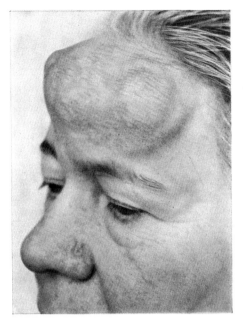

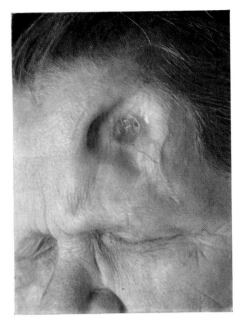

878   Late benign syphilis
Two indolent gummas of the forehead
arising from the periosteum. Perforation is imminent and will result in
sharply circumscribed punched-out
ulcers.

879   Late benign syphilis
Gumma of the forehead, drained and
largely healed, leaving osseous defect.

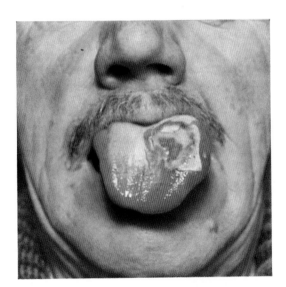

880   Late benign syphilis
Ulcerated gumma of the tongue. Punched-out, deep ulcer
on the left side of the tongue. Differentiation from carcinoma
associated with leukoplakia is important.

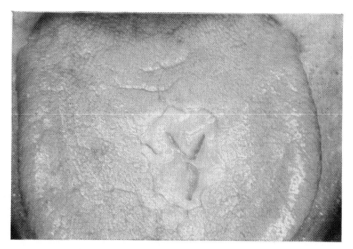

881 Late benign syphilis
Gumma of the tongue.

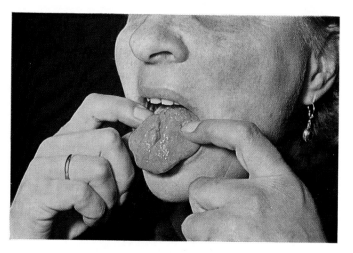

882 Late benign syphilis
Gumma of the tongue.

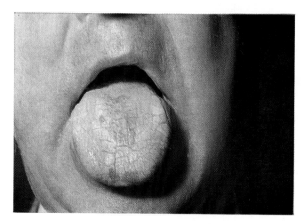

883 Late benign syphilis
Syphilitic leukoplakia of the tongue. Surface of the
tongue is porcelain-colored and shows characteristic
pattern.

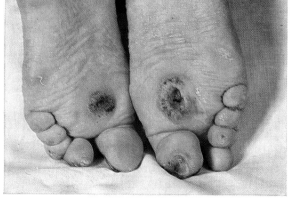

884 Neurosyphilis
Malum perforans in tabes dorsalis.

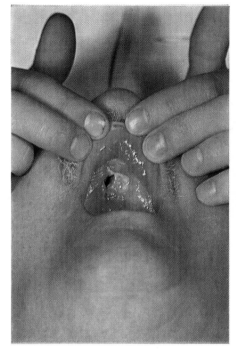

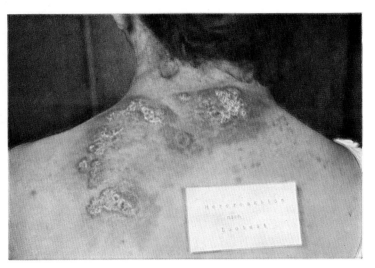

885 Late benign syphilis
Perforating ulcer of the hard palate.
Similar ulcers may be caused by tuberculosis, carcinoma, dental fistulas,
osteomyelitis, following scarlet or ty-
phoid fever, blastomycosis, or congenital deformities.

886 Late benign syphilis
Flare up of tuberoserpiginous syphilis following intracutaneous injection of Luotest. This test is positive in
late benign syphilis of the skin and in late congenital syphilis.
It is negative in early syphilis, and cardiovascular and
neurosyphilis.

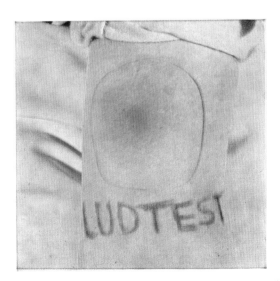

887 Positive Luotest reaction

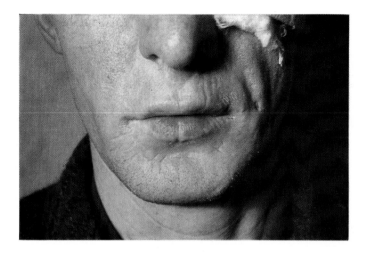

888   Congenital syphilis

Syphilitic rhagades (PARROT's lines). Radial linear scars about the mouth
produced by perioral infiltrative syphilids in early life.

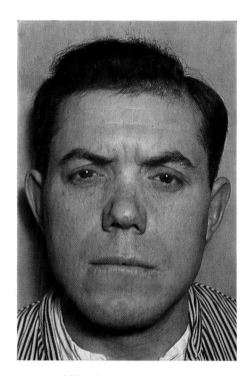

889   Congenital syphilis

Saddle nose is another permanent stigma produced by congenital
syphilis. A diagnostic sign, especially when seen in association with
PARROT's lines.

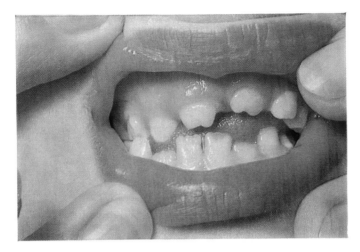

890 Congenital syphilis

HUTCHINSON's teeth. The upper central incisors of the second dentition show characteristic peg shape and central notching; the adjacent teeth are also deformed. Such dentition is diagnostic for congenital syphilis, especially when associated with diffuse interstitial keratitis and deafness (HUTCHINSON's triad).

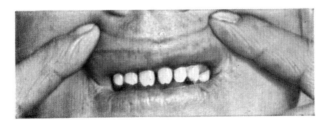

891 Congenital syphilis
HUTCHINSON's teeth.

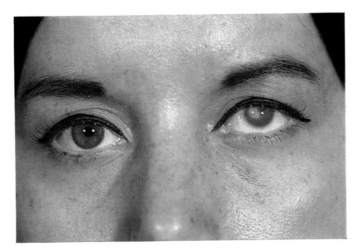

892 Congenital syphilis
Diffuse interstitial keratitis of the left eye.

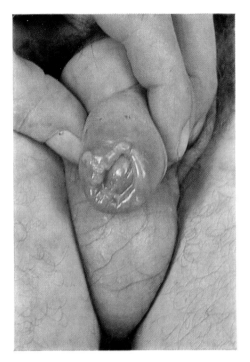

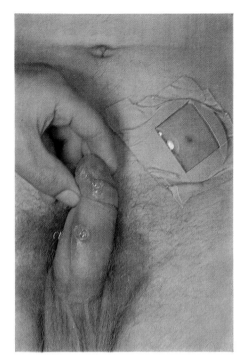

893 Chancroid (ulcus molle)

Multiple tender, soft, purulent ulcerations surrounded by erythematous, edematous skin.

894 Chancroid (ulcus molle)

Soft, tender, purulent ulcers with erythematous, ragged, undermined borders. Regional lymphadenopathy. Inoculation of tissue fragments into the abdominal wall produced a new chancroid lesion after two days.

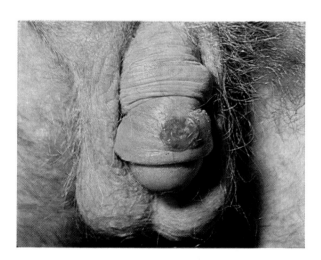

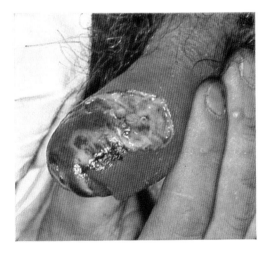

895 Chancroid (ulcus molle)

Elevated variety. Soft, tender ulcer with granulomatous tissue raised above the level of the surrounding skin.

896 Chancroid (ulcus molle)

Gangrenous form with rapid degeneration of ulcers due to mixed infection.

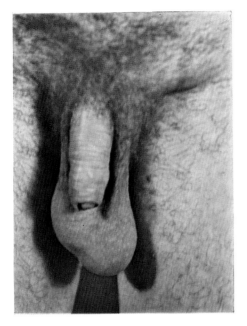

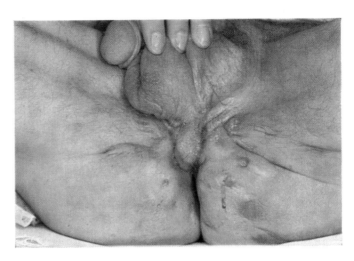

897 Lymphogranuloma venereum
Inconspicuous primary lesion with
unilateral lymphadenopathy.

898 Lymphogranuloma venerum
Anorectal ulcers.

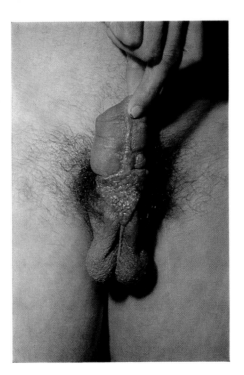

899 Granuloma inguinale
Sharply defined, indolent, raised, granulomatous,
ulcerative lesions with fetid discharge.

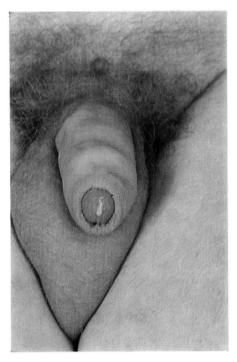

900　Gonorrheal urethritis
Creamy purulent discharge
from the urethra.

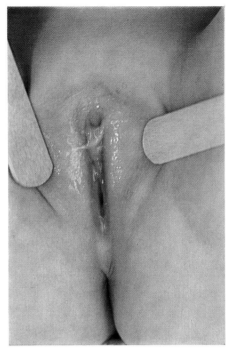

901　Gonorrheal vulvovaginitis in infancy
Edema, erythema, and purulent discharge from the vagina, vestibulum, urethral orifice, and labia majora and minora.

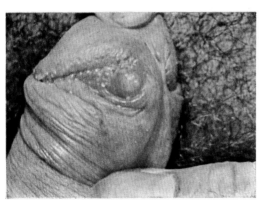

902　Gonorrheal abscess
Of parafrenular area shortly before perforation. Differentiated from chancroid by smears stained for gonococci.

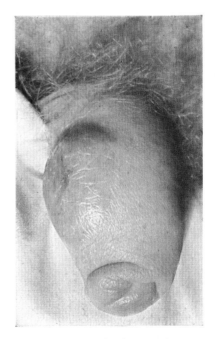

903　Gonorrheal cavernitis
Shortly before perforation.
Involving urethral corpus
cavernosum only.

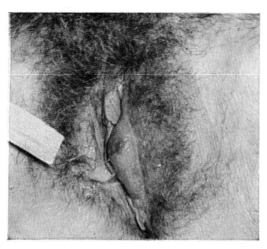

904 Gonorrheal bartholinitis
Acute lesion shortly before perforation.
Differentiated from folliculitis or furuncle
by bacterial smear.

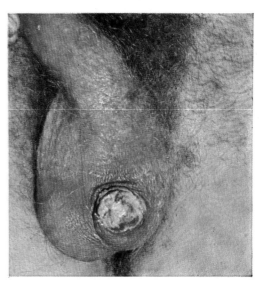

905 Gonorrheal gangrene
Testicular gangrene; a rare complication of
gonorrhea.

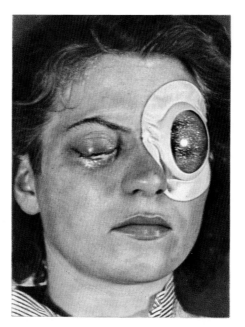

906 Gonorrhea of eye (gonoblennorrhea)
Severe inflammatory edema of both eyelids and purulent
conjunctivitis due to accidental contamination with gonorrheal pus.

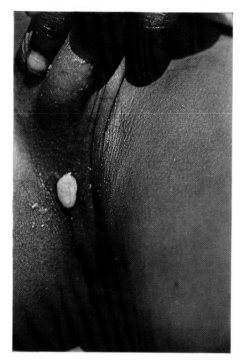

907 Yaws, primary stage

Primary lesion at the portal of entry of
Treponema pertenue.

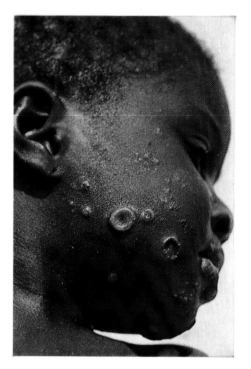

908 Yaws, secondary stage

Crusted papular exanthema with lesions of
varying size, some in annular configuration.
Typically, the lips are also involved.

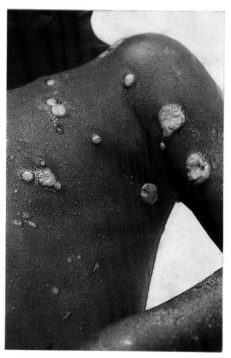

909 Yaws, secondary stage

Same patient as shown in figure 908, showing
similar lesions on the trunk and extremities.

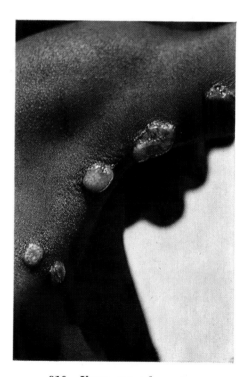

910 Yaws, secondary stage

Raspberry-like, superficially eroded, and granulomatous papillomas of the posterior axillary fold.

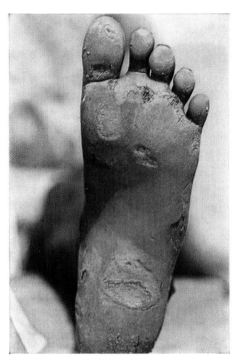

911 Yaws, secondary stage

Hyperkeratotic, scaling papular lesions of the sole.

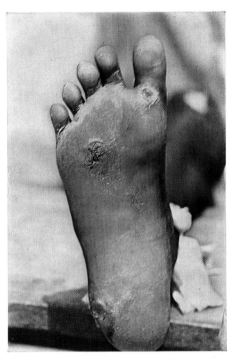

912 Yaws, secondary stage

Ulcerations or large hyperkeratotic lesions resembling plantar warts are sometimes seen beside hyperkeratotic and scaling plantar lesions (see figure 911).

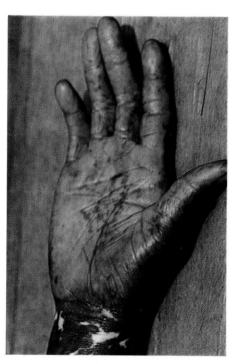

913 Yaws, secondary stage

Contractures of third, fourth and fifth fingers. Healed lesions often leave patchy depigmentation.

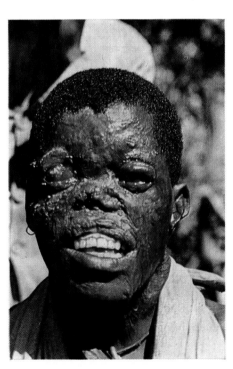

914 Yaws, late stage

Gangosa (rhinopharyngitis mutilans) with severe destruction of soft tissues and bones.

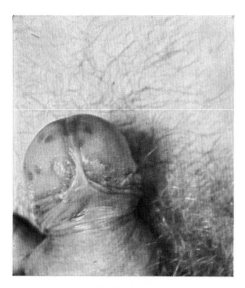

915 Balanitis

Erosive circinate lesions. Pinhead-sized, whitish macerations develop into larger lesions with central erosions, and finally coalesce to form circinate configurations or geographic patterns. There is a thin, fetid, purulent discharge due to mixed infection.

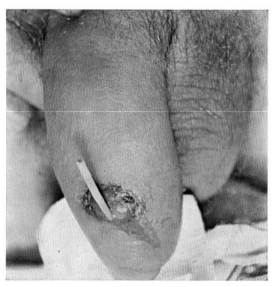

916 Balanitis

Gangrenous form with perforation of the foreskin. This disorder may occur alone or in association with chancroid, producing gangrenous chancroid.

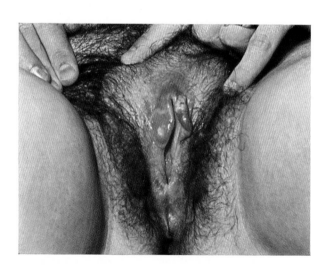

917 Ulcus vulvae acutum (LIPSCHÜTZ)

Rapidly growing ulcer on the internal aspect of the labium minus, more common in young girls and virginal young women. Causative organism is the otherwise saprophytic Bacillus crassus.

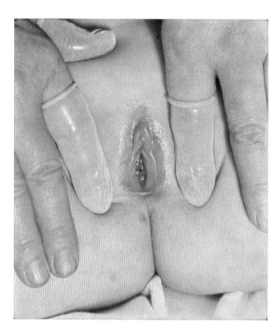

918 Diphtheritic vulvitis

Although the most common type of inflammation and discharge from the external genitals of prepubertal girls is due to gonorrhea, the rare diphtheric infection of the vulva produces similar changes.

Diseases of the Tongue

Enanthemas and changes of the oral mucosa associated with various dermatoses have been discussed in the respective chapters. The following remain to be mentioned:

Leukoplakia

Granulomatous inflammatory diseases (e.g., syphilis), chemical agents (tar products in cigarette smoke, arsenic), or physical irritants (galvanic and thermal) may be responsible for keratinization of the oral mucosa, which is sometimes followed by cancerous degeneration.

Plummer-Vinson Syndrome

Glossitis, dysphagia, and perlèche may occur as a result of iron deficiency anemia.

"Antibiotic tongue"

During tetracycline treatment the mucosa of the tongue often assumes a smooth, atrophic, inflamed, reddened appearance.

Black hairy tongue

This condition may follow antibiotic therapy. Vitamin deficiency may be an important etiologic factor. The discoloration may be black, yellowish-brown, or bluish-green.

Lingua plicata
(Furrowed tongue; Scrotal tongue)

This relatively frequent change of the surface of the tongue is harmless, but may invite bacterial invasion.

Geographic tongue

Circumscribed irregular, smooth, red areas are characteristic of this disease of the mucous membrane of the tongue. Desquamation is more pronounced in the central portions of the lesions. The plaques spread toward the periphery, thus creating a rapidly changing pattern.

Glossitis rhombica mediana
(Brocq-Pautrier)

This is a benign disease, characterized by a red rhomboid plaque in the dorsal midline of the tongue.

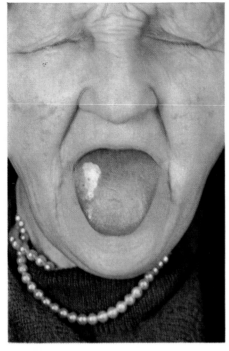

919   Leukoplakia of the tongue
Syphilitic inflammation could not be demonstrated in this case.

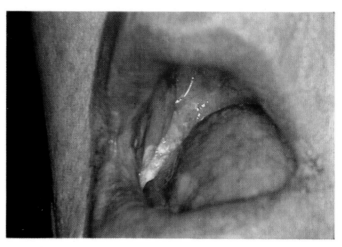

920   Leukoplakia of the tongue and buccal mucosa
Marked whitish discoloration. Etiology unknown.

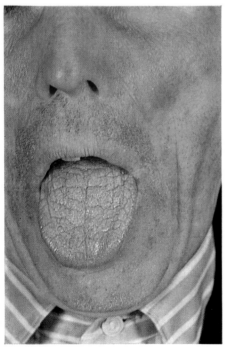

921

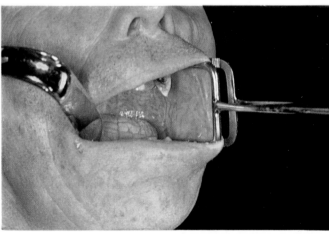

922

921 and 922   Smokers' patches (leukokeratosis nicotinica)
On the tongue and oral mucosa. Characteristic square or polygonal, white thickened patches.

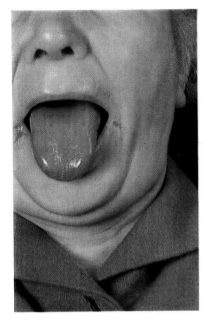

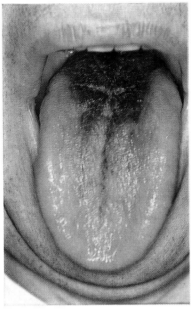

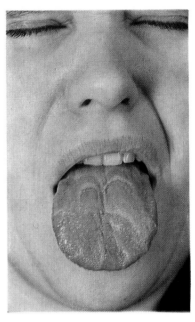

923 Plummer-Vinson syndrome
Smooth, atrophic, red tongue with perlèche of corners of the mouth in an anemic patient.

924 Black hairy tongue
Of unknown origin. Hyperplastic changes of the filiform papillae.

925 Geographic tongue
Irregular, circumscribed, red, desquamative lesions in central portion of the tongue.

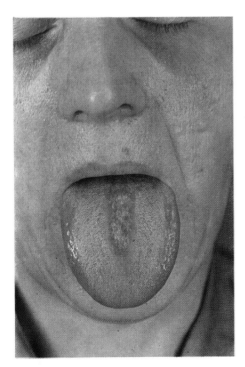

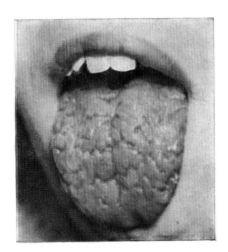

926 Glossitis rhombica mediana
Band-like, relatively large lesion without papillae in midline of the tongue.

927 Lingua plicata (furrowed tongue)
Symmetrical arrangement of furrows, resembling the veins of a leaf.

Index

Numbers in **bold face type** indicate pages on which illustrations appear.